IS THERE A DOCTOR IN THE HOUSE?

IS THERE A DOCTOR IN THE HOUSE?

*Market Signals and
Tomorrow's Supply of Doctors*

RICHARD M. SCHEFFLER

STANFORD GENERAL BOOKS

*An imprint of Stanford University Press
Stanford, California*

Stanford University Press
Stanford, California

©2008 by the Board of Trustees of the Leland Stanford Junior University.
All rights reserved.

Printed in the United States of America on acid-free, archival-quality paper

Library of Congress Cataloging-in-Publication Data

Scheffler, Richard M.
  Is there a doctor in the house? : market signals and tomorrow's supply of doc-
tors / Richard M. Scheffler.
      p. cm.
  Includes bibliographical references and index.
  ISBN 978-0-8047-0032-0 (cloth : alk. paper)
  1. Physicians--Supply and demand--United States. 2. Physicians--Supply and
demand--Forecasting. 3. Managed care plans (Medical care)--United States. 4.
Managed care plans (Medical care)--United States--Finance. 5. Medical care,
Cost of--United States. 6. Medical education--United States--Finance. I. Title.
  RA410.7.S34 2008
  338.4'761092--dc22   2008024424

Typeset at Stanford University Press in 10.5/15 Minion

This book is dedicated to the incredible physicians who have taken care of me and who serve society day after day. I understand on a personal level the value of what these dedicated individuals do.

And to my seventeen-year-old son, Zach, who continually inspires me with his curiosity. I recognize that kind of eagerness to know as the lifeblood of human efforts to expand the literature in any field of inquiry.

CONTENTS

Acknowledgments   xi

PART I   **MARKET POWER AND THE
          DOCTOR SUPPLY**

Chapter 1   The Supply Cycle of Doctors   3

Chapter 2   Managed Care Redistributes Market Power   18

Chapter 3   Physician Incomes: Following the Money   28

Chapter 4   Who Are the Doctors, and Where Are They?   43

Chapter 5   Reshaping the Workforce: Nurse Practitioners
              and Physician Assistants   53

Chapter 6   Doctor Supply Forecasts: More or Less   64

Chapter 7   The "Right" Number of Doctors in a Better
              Health Care System   75

PART II   **CONVERSATIONS WITH THE EXPERTS**

          Toward Tiered High-Performance Networks
          Alain C. Enthoven, Stanford University   95

          Primary Care and the Medical Home
          Karen Davis, The Commonwealth Fund   100

Rethinking the Financing of GME
Gail Wilensky, Project HOPE   104

What the Market Signals Are Saying
Mark V. Pauly, University of Pennsylvania   107

Residents, Payment, and the Global Market
Joseph P. Newhouse, Harvard University   110

Physician Income and the Potential of P4P
Uwe E. Reinhardt, Princeton University   112

Measuring Performance: How and Why
Peter R. Carroll, University of California, San Francisco   116

Paying for Primary Care in an Outmoded System
Jordan J. Cohen, Arnold P. Gold Foundation   120

Advanced-Practice Clinicians Challenge
Traditional Model
*Tracey O. Fremd, California Association for
Nurse Practitioners*   123

Chronic Care Models and Turf Battles
Gary Gitnick, University of California, Los Angeles   127

Free Medical Education—with Strings
Donald Goldmann, Institute for Healthcare Improvement   129

Understanding the Real Cost of Medical Education
Atul Grover, Association of American Medical Colleges   132

Primary Care: How Much Does Money Matter?
Kevin Grumbach, University of California, San Francisco   135

A Regional Approach to Health Disparities
Risa Lavizzo-Mourey, Robert Wood Johnson Foundation   137

A Short History of Medical Education and Diversity
Philip R. Lee, Stanford University   140

Too Many Doctors, Too Little Efficiency
Arnold Milstein, William M. Mercer   143

Taking Responsibility for Generating
America's Doctors
Fitzhugh Mullan, George Washington University   149

We Expect Too Much from Physicians
Edward O'Neil, University of California, San Francisco   154

The Integrated System: Paying for Primary Care
Robert Pearl, Kaiser Permanente   157

The Declining Role of Government:
It's Time to Prepare
Philip A. Pizzo, Stanford University   161

Tomorrow's Doctors Want Something Different
*Edward S. Salsberg, Association of American
   Medical Colleges*   164

The Medical Home and Other Ways
to Save Primary Care
Steven Schroeder, University of California, San Francisco   168

External Reporting and Other Keys to P4P
Stephen M. Shortell, University of California, Berkeley   172

What the Business Model
and the Military Model Know
Mark D. Smith, California HealthCare Foundation   175

More Doctors Does Not Equal Better Outcomes
*John E. Wennberg, Dartmouth Institute for Health Policy
   and Clinical Practice*   180

Doctors as Team Players
*William J. Barcellona, California Association of
   Physician Groups*   184

Doctors: Stop Being Depressed and
Redesign the System
Ian Morrison, Institute for the Future   186

A Final Word   191

Appendix A:
The Cost of Training a Doctor and the Return on Investment   **201**

Appendix B:
Methodology for Forecasting Doctor Shortages   **213**

Notes   **217**

Index   **233**

ACKNOWLEDGMENTS

This book is the product of many hands. I would first like to thank my doctoral students, several of whom contributed to the research for this book while they worked with me at The Nicholas C. Petris Center on Health Care Markets & Consumer Welfare. A few stand out for particular recognition. Brian Quinn gathered comprehensive background information and brought me up to speed with a concept paper on managed care. Nona Kocher made a significant contribution by tirelessly finding material for me, including data that were not easily accessible. Jenny Liu contributed in a variety of ways, not only helping me with the empirical analysis but serving as my "professor" by offering very thoughtful ideas on how the book should take shape. Ashley Hodgson, studying for a Ph.D. in economics, served as a sounding board for my economic analysis and also did empirical work. She helped correct all my ambiguities and mistakes.

I want especially to thank several people who did important reviews of the manuscript.

David Mechanic, Ph.D., is the René Dubos University Professor of Behavioral Sciences and director of the Institute for Health, Health Care Policy, and Aging Research at Rutgers University. David read the manuscript carefully and provided incredibly detailed and insightful comments.

Paul Feldstein, Ph.D., is a professor and Robert Gumbiner Chair in Health Care Management, Graduate School of Management, University of California, Irvine. He gave me some sense of balance in looking at both the market and the policy sides of the issues.

Mark Pauly, Ph.D., is a professor, vice dean, and chair of the Health Care Systems Department in the Wharton School, University of Pennsylvania. He gave me comments from his deep knowledge of the intricacies of the health care market.

I am grateful to Stephen M. Shortell, Ph.D., who encouraged me to write this book and gave me the time needed to work on it. He is the Blue Cross of California Distinguished Professor of Health Policy and Management and a professor of organization behavior in the School of Public Health and the Haas School of Business at the University of California, Berkeley. He is also the dean of the School of Public Health at Berkeley.

My colleague William H. Dow, Ph.D., is an associate professor of economics in the School of Public Health at the University of California, Berkeley. I am grateful for his rigorous attention to detail, policy knowledge, and quantitative insights.

My old friend Julian Legrand, Ph.D., is the Richard Titmuss Professor of Social Policy at the London School of Economics. He offered valuable comments from the other side of the Atlantic.

Roger Feldman, Ph.D., is the Blue Cross Professor of Health Insurance and professor of economics, University of Minnesota. He is my friend and former colleague from our days at the University of North Carolina at Chapel Hill, when we were both real economists in the Economics Department. He was kind enough to give me insightful comments on the estimates of the costs of medical education included in this book.

My dear colleague and longtime friend Teh-Wei Hu, Ph.D., professor emeritus of Health Economics in the School of Public Health at the University of California, Berkeley, did his best to make sure I got the numbers right.

Cheryl Cashin, Ph.D., is an economist and a postdoctoral fellow at the Petris Center. John Friedman, Ph.D., is a Robert Wood Johnson Foundation Scholar in Health Policy in the School of Public Health at the University of California, Berkeley. They not only made important comments on the manuscript but were willing to have intense discussions about portions of the book that needed clarity and improvement.

The Petris Center staff has my gratitude. In particular, Timothy Brown, associate director, gave me important feedback. Some of the research we did at the Petris Center served as input for the book. Other staff members who put in valuable time and effort are James Ross, manager of finance and administration; Brent Fulton, health researcher; Amy Nuttbrock, program coordinator; Jessica Lubniewski, executive assistant; Stephanie Hastrup, executive assistant; and Candy Pareja, research coordinator.

Financial support and encouragement came from two foundation heads. Steven Schroeder, M.D., is Distinguished Professor of Health and Health Care, Division of General Internal Medicine, Department of Medicine, at the University of California, San Francisco. A former president and CEO of the Robert Wood Johnson Foundation, he gave me a presidential grant to allow me to do some pilot work for the book. Dan M. Fox, Ph.D., former president of the Milbank Memorial Fund, also financially supported me, and encouraged me to think deeply about issues of public policy and to write a book that would inform policymakers at the state and federal levels.

At the end of the day, I want to thank Susan Anthony, senior editor at Petris, who helped me find my voice as a writer. This was not an easy task, as I have been accustomed to writing research papers. She not only edited my work but made sense of it. This book is in many ways a joint effort.

My deepest gratitude goes to the twenty-seven individuals—leading figures in academic medicine, health economics, and health policy—who were willing to talk to me in depth about the broad implications of these subjects. I was inspired by their knowledge and passion. To a person, they provided insights that measurably enriched these pages.

I

MARKET POWER AND THE DOCTOR SUPPLY

1

THE SUPPLY CYCLE OF DOCTORS

OF DOCTORS AND RESTAURANTS

Currently we have almost nine hundred thousand actively practicing physicians in the United States. Many experts say this is an oversupply.[1] Yet how can there be too many physicians when we typically must wait weeks or more to get an appointment with our doctor?

One way to demystify this paradox is to consider the city of San Francisco. This medium-size city is unique for a number of reasons, two of which are its high ratios of both physicians and restaurants per capita. In fact, it has been ranked the top American city on both measures.[2]

So let us briefly talk about food, for which San Francisco is famous. Excellent restaurants help attract some sixteen million tourists to the city annually.[3] Many of these visitors phone the best-known restaurants—maybe a dozen or more—only to find they have to wait several weeks for a reservation. Should they conclude there aren't enough restaurants in San Francisco?

I wanted to see if there were similarities in getting access to popular restaurants and doctors, so my team and I conducted some informal research.

We called restaurants that were listed in the Zagat Survey guide[4] as the most popular and that served the best food and asked for a reservation for four people for the next available Saturday night. The average wait time was forty-one days. For comparison, we also called restaurants picked randomly from the phone book. We called on a Thursday, and in every case, we were given a reservation for the next Saturday.

The phenomenon at work is that everybody is competing to go to the top twenty restaurants, resulting in long wait lists for reservations. As most of these disappointed tourists discover, there are excellent restaurants around practically every corner in San Francisco, and a surprising number of them don't even require a reservation.

To look at access to doctors, we called physicians from *San Francisco Magazine*'s "Best Doctors 2005: The Bay Area's 520 Top Docs."[5] This listing was created by Best Doctors, Inc., which "asked the country's most respected physicians a simple question: Who would you send your loved ones to?" Our research team used the list to call for a nonurgent routine visit with a primary care doctor, and also called a similar number of doctors picked at random from the phone book. The average wait time was sixty-six days for a doctor on the "Top Docs" list, and twenty-seven days for doctors randomly selected.[6]

As with restaurants, a similar mechanism is at work when people arrange to get medical care for a particular problem. Most people are calling the same doctors in very much the way they call the same set of restaurants. And they find that the wait time for an appointment is similarly lengthy. But this does not indicate a shortage of doctors in San Francisco; in fact, it's very much the opposite.[7] Clearly there is more to this story.[8]

Others have looked at physician appointment wait times. In their 2004 survey, Merritt, Hawkins & Associates examined wait times in fifteen American cities for first-time appointments with four types of specialists: cardiologists, dermatologists, ob/gyns, and orthopedic surgeons (see Table 1.1). The results varied greatly by city. In cardiology, for example, the average wait in Seattle was only nine days, whereas in Boston it was thirty-seven days. To see a dermatologist in New York would take nine days, whereas in Boston the wait would average fifty days. The wait for an ob/gyn appointment in Miami would be ten days, whereas the wait in Boston would be forty-five days. In fact, Boston reported the longest average wait times in three of the four specialties surveyed, and the second-longest wait in the remaining specialty (orthopedic surgery).[9] What's going on? Boston is home to some of the most prestigious medical schools and teaching hospitals in the world. This fact may be at the heart of the wait time problem (although managed care and malpractice rates may affect physician retention): people want to go to the best doctors and believe that Boston offers the best.

For a fuller understanding of the adequacy of the supply of doctors, we must expand our view to include rural and inner-city areas. Even in a greater metropolitan region that has a healthy supply of doctors, some areas will not have enough. This raises the question of the difference between *supply* and *distribution*, which can be illuminated with another example involving the quest for a meal. Suppose ten friends arrive at a dinner party at your house, where the table is set with ten plates of food. Ten chairs are evenly spaced around the table, but most of the plates are grouped around just seven of them. Three of your guests end up with two plates of food each, four guests each have a single plate, and three guests go home hungry. This is a distribution problem, a fundamental component of the physician supply challenge in the United States.

Table 1.1. Average wait times in days in 2004, by metropolitan area

City	Cardiology		Dermatology		OB/Gyn		Orthopedic Surgery	
	Wait time	MDs per cap	Wait time	MDs per cap	Wait time	MDs per cap	Wait time	MDs per cap
Los Angeles	14	7.1	14	4.1	19	13.7	43	7.8
San Diego	17	6.9	12	5.9	31	11.7	13	10.1
Denver	23	15.4	21	5.9	23	31.2	23	15.4
Washington, D.C.	12	18.4	15	10.3	11	34.5	8	19.3
Miami	21	12.3	17	5.9	10	13.1	11	8.1
Seattle	9	9.3	27	6.1	26	15.9	12	12.6
Atlanta	17	14	21	10.7	24	37.6	8	16.5
Boston	37	36.3	50	11.3	45	29.4	24	26.9
Detroit	20	4.9	25	2.9	39	11.9	18	3.7
Minneapolis	15	11.8	43	6.2	20	19.4	19	14
New York	22	33.5	9	23	14	45.6	16	30.3
Portland	25	8.8	30	7.4	30	22.6	19	11.9
Philadelphia	27	14.4	33	5.4	28	18.4	18	11.8
Dallas	10	8.1	34	3.8	17	16.5	10	8.2
Houston	11	8.9	13	4.1	20	13.3	15	7.8
Weighted average	18.8	10.6	24.3	6	23.3	17.4	16.9	10.6

SOURCES: Average wait times are obtained from Merritt, Hawkins & Associates, "Summary Report: 2004 Survey of Physician Appointment Wait Times," www.merritthawkins.com/pdf/Survey_2004_Patient_Wait_Times.pdf. Data on physicians and population are obtained from the Area Resource File, 2005.

WHY WE NEED TO GET IT RIGHT

The supply of doctors is crucial to health because physicians are the lynchpin of the medical system and have enormous influence on the quality of health care and the health status of all of us. Doctors are considered a "social good" because the health of the population affects the productivity of the economy and the well-being of everyone in it.

For individuals, the crucial question is this: *Can I see a doctor—a good doctor—when I need one?* This is the square one of the health care system for most people.

Although restaurant supply is determined entirely in the marketplace, the doctor supply is strongly influenced by the government. Not only does it subsidize the training of doctors, it enables large numbers of international medical graduates to be trained in the United States and often to go on to practice here.

What would happen if Americans suddenly started visiting doctors more often? This is not entirely hypothetical; if health insurance programs are expanded, that is exactly what would happen. An aging population or changing disease levels could also lead to a sudden increase in patient visits and need for services. How can doctors respond? The main avenue open to them is to increase the number of hours they work—but only to the point beyond which they would consider it to be unreasonable. After that threshold, they might discourage additional patients and visits by raising their prices. This is what we mean by a physician "shortage."

A *shortage*, as health economists use the term, does not mean that there are people who want service and are not getting it. Rather, the price rises until the extra people waiting in line no longer want the service. It's too expensive for them. Everyone who wants service at the new, higher price is getting it. That's how markets work. This is how they "clear," even in the shortage situation.

The same market-clearing situation occurs in a surplus. If people stop going to the doctor as often, doctors will be waiting around their offices for patients to show up. We may, then, have a case in which five doctors are doing the work that could be done by four. What's wrong with that? It's too wasteful. It costs society about $1 million to train a doctor[10] (see Appendix A for details). We can't afford to waste *any* of this extremely valuable health workforce.

And there is another deleterious impact of oversupply. It sets up potential health hazards as more doctors are forced to compete for the same patients. Some may feel compelled to provide services that are marginally beneficial in order to maintain their incomes and keep their practices going.[11] Oversupply creates an incentive for doctors to perform services for which they may have little experience. If they don't have enough patients, they can gain by performing tasks on their current patients that they would otherwise refer to a specialist. And with relatively few patients to treat, they have fewer opportunities to gain the needed experience in specialized procedures or services. It is well-established that, in medicine, practice makes perfect in terms of health outcomes.[12]

How, then, do we know when we have the "right" number of doctors? If the current supply can reasonably adjust their hours, either up or down, to take care of all the patients who walk in the door, then we have the most efficient number. If doctors cannot reasonably adjust their hours, unnecessary inefficiencies arise. Either prices rise too quickly or doctors wait around. That's inefficient even in a market-clearing situation.

Of course, other forces can affect the supply of services. If physician productivity improves, then the same doctor can provide more services without increasing hours. Productivity can be improved by adding more nurse practitioners or physician assistants, by training the doctor to use new information technology, and by working in teams. Productivity changes generally happen slowly, however. Clearly productivity improvements will be more efficient than training new doctors. The real question is, How much more productivity can we reasonably get out of doctors?

It is also worth noting that the government plays a major role as both a buyer of services and a regulator of prices. The government sets a fixed schedule of prices it will pay for particular services that Medicare patients need. Doctors can either accept or reject these patients. Doctors often take Medicare patients in addition to participating in the private market already described. However, the Medicare price schedule depends in part on market conditions in the private market, so the two are intertwined. The price schedule for Medicaid is lower than for Medicare, so fewer physicians accept Medicaid patients.

HOW DO WE KNOW WHERE WE STAND?

How do we know if we are in the middle of a doctor shortage? Physicians do not generally record the number of hours they work, and even if they did, it wouldn't be known what the average doctor considers to be a "reasonable" work schedule.

Market signals cannot tell us if we are moving toward an equilibrium[13] or away from it unless we have a benchmark—a point in time when there was the "right" number of doctors. As a starting point, I propose that this happened sometime around the 1980s. Economists and policy experts in the early to mid-1990s were projecting physician surpluses. This was pretty much true across the board. Continuing along the same line of thinking, the Balanced Budget Act of 1997 limited the number of resident physicians that Medicare was willing to finance. Policymakers basically believed at that point that the country didn't need to be producing as many doctors as it was.

Then, in 2006, the Association of American Medical Colleges (AAMC) put out a report crying for help in the wake of what it deemed to be an impending shortage of doctors.[14] What had changed? If the policymakers are reasonably accurate in their forecasting techniques, this indicates that there was an equilibrium some time in between the surplus forecasts and the shortage forecasts. For this reason, I assume that somewhere around the year 2000, America had the right number of doctors. This benchmark is also consistent with the fact that physician incomes were not moving very much around this time period. It isn't a perfect baseline, but from a policy perspective, I believe it's the best benchmark we have to work with.

Given our baseline, we need some way of assessing where the market for doctors is heading. This brings me to the main purpose of this book. When we look into the future, we have two things to think about: trends and turning points. Some people view turning points as random occurrences—shocks that come out of left field and are impossible to prepare for. As an economist and policy analyst, I like to think differently. Turning points generally happen when pressure builds up and forces a shift, such as a change in the structure of the market.

History can educate us about turning points in the supply of doctors. For instance, an oversupply of doctors some thirty years ago caused a build-up in pressure. This resulted in managed care infiltrating the market to relieve some of those pressures. In essence, managed care took market power out of the hands of doctors, who had been using their power to induce demand and raise prices. Payers and consumers were no longer willing to go along with that, and managed care stepped in to curb the "rents"[15] that doctors were enjoying. Managed care firms encouraged the use of less expensive labor, such as nurse practitioners and physician assistants, to do things that doctors did at a higher price. Managed care has, of course, introduced new issues, which I will go into in some detail in later chapters. The main point that I am making here is that pressure builds up in a market and calls for a restructuring. This is when turning points emerge. Policymakers need to be on the lookout for key turning points in an industry, or they could greatly miss the mark when they make decisions.

In order to be sensitive to areas in which there may be a turning point, we have to know where there is pressure in the market. That's where market signals come in. Doctor incomes, economic rates of return on training, the number of doctors in different specialties, and the spatial distribution of doctors—all of these give market signals. For example, doctor salaries have not risen as fast as salaries in other professions in recent years. During this time, the number of nonphysician workers in the health care sector has risen rapidly, while the number of doctors has grown only modestly. These facts together indicate that there has been a greater amount of substitution going on. Nurse practitioners, nurses, and other personnel have taken on tasks that the physician used to do. This has relieved some of the demand on physicians and made each more efficient. By looking at the various market indicators, then, we can piece together a picture of the situation today and going forward.

Market indicators can do a lot. They can identify places where market pressure might push the market in a different direction. They can also help to project trends into the future. Economic models help us tell where the market is going if there isn't a turning point. Market indicators suggest a baseline point for thinking about where we are going. To begin, let us see what the past can tell us about the structure of the industry and how built-up pressure leads to change.

A NEW VIEW: THE PHYSICIAN SUPPLY CYCLE

If we are to move toward the right number of doctors, we must first consider what is meant by "right." There are schools of thought on this matter, as I will discuss in later chapters. My premise is that the supply and demand of doctors are best understood in the framework of a market. And I further posit that the emergence of managed care beginning in the 1980s "connected" what had been a disconnected or inefficient market. Though far from perfect, the market forced doctors to compete on price in order to enter the managed care environment. The most telling evidence of this dramatic change can be observed through physician incomes, as I will examine in detail in Chapter 3. Another result of the market shift has been the strong emergence of physician assistants and nurse practitioners, which changed the size and character of the physician workforce.

These changes did not occur in a vacuum. To understand the way the doctor supply and demand have evolved in the United States, we must consider some landmark events that influenced them. Many health industry observers have dutifully compiled the historical record on physician supply. The depiction in Figure 1.1 highlights a number of markers that are significant to the *market* view of physician supply, and subjects them to fuller examination from this perspective.[16]

These historical landmarks tell a story about the marketplace for physicians that I call the Supply Cycle of Doctors. To see the pattern emerge, I will analyze the steps along the way.

Doctor Shortage

The story begins with a perceived doctor shortage. From 1900 to the mid-1960s, there was almost universal agreement that the nation did not have enough physicians, even though the per capita supply remained relatively stable. Nevertheless, the perception of shortage influenced the events that followed. I use the term *perceived shortage* because there wasn't any real way of knowing, nor were any studies conducted with acceptable analytic rigor. However, a report published in 1910 found that medical schools did not base their training on a high enough standard of science.[17] The publication of this report resulted in the closure of many medical schools, and this in turn caused the number of medical graduates per year to drop precipitously.

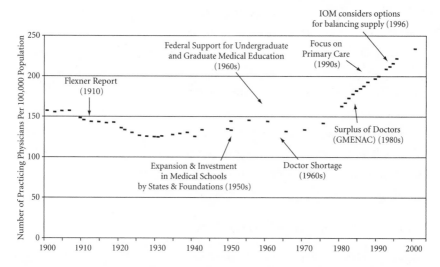

Figure 1.1. Physician workforce milestones in the twenty-first century, 1900–2000

SOURCES: *Historical Statistics of the United States—Colonial Times to 1970*, U.S. Department of Commerce, 1975; *Physician Characteristics and Distribution in the U.S.*, 2001–2001 Edition, American Medical Association; and *Physician Characteristics and Distribution in the U.S.*, 2005 Edition, American Medical Association.

Doctor Supply Build-Up

Now fast forward to the 1950s and 1960s, when anecdotal evidence from the previous decades led to a general consensus that the United States had a shortage of physicians,[18] prompting the federal and state governments to allocate funds to increase the supply.[19] This support began around 1963, and by 1976 had resulted in the building of some forty new medical schools and the expansion of many older ones.[20]

A signal event was the passage of Medicare and Medicaid in 1965. This was a directional change for the nation because, for the first time, the federal government took on the responsibility of providing health care for the elderly and disabled. These two programs enabled more Americans to seek and receive health care, which subsequently increased the demand for physicians.[21]

It must be noted that Medicare was not created because of concern about the supply of doctors. It was a mechanism to fund hospitals, whose primary users were the elderly and disabled—the typical Medicare population. Government dollars were allocated to the education of medical residents, which took place in hospitals, triggering a sharp increase in the supply of doctors.[22]

Medicare was only using residency programs as a mechanism to channel funding to the elderly and disabled. The expansion of residency programs was a secondary, and arguably unintentional, consequence. This unintentional policy of financing graduate medical education still exists. By funding residency training, Medicare increased the supply of doctors.[23]

Medicare boosted the supply of physicians and helped cause a jump in the proportion of doctors who were specialists.[24] Between 1965 and 1980, as medical schools continued to grow, the number of actively practicing doctors per 100,000 population increased from 132 to 163.[25] The growth in health care expenditures during that same time span was startling.

Doctor Oversupply Spurs Competition

Finally, in 1980, the government began to take notice. Various commissions and studies all pointed to a current and future oversupply of physicians in the nation. Figure 1.2 summarizes these estimates. The Graduate Medical Educa-

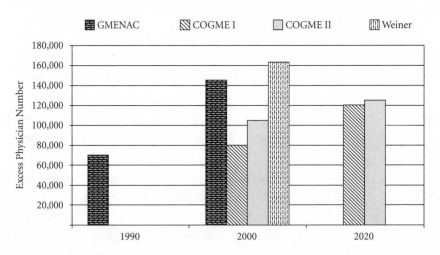

Figure 1.2. Various forecasts of physician oversupply

SOURCES: Graduate Medical Education National Advisory Committee (GMENAC), *Report to the Secretary: Dept. of Health and Human Services. Vol. 1, Summary Report,* DHHS Publication No. (HRA) 81-651, Washington, DC: Health Resources Administration, 1986; Council on Graduate Medical Education, *COGME (I) 1994 Recommendations to Improve Access to Health Care Through Physician Workforce Reform,* Rockville, MD: U.S. Dept. of Health and Human Services, 1994; *COGME (II) 1995 Physician Workforce Funding Recommendations for Department of Health and Human Services' Programs,* Council on Graduate Medical Education, 7th Report, Rockville, MD: U.S. Dept. of Health and Human Services, 1995; J. P. Weiner, "Forecasting the Effects of Health Reform on U.S. Physician Workforce Requirement: Evidence from HMO Staffing Patterns," *Journal of the American Medical Association* 272, no. 3 (July 20, 1994): 222–230.

tion National Advisory Committee (GMENAC) warned that by 1990, the nation would have seventy thousand more physicians than needed.[26] Numerous government reports and significant papers were published in the 1990s that suggested even larger surpluses in 2000 and 2020.[27]

Managed Care Growth

Enter managed care. Managed care is an arrangement that shifts power away from doctors to payers. For example, managed care contracts place limits on services, whereas fee-for-service reimburses whatever the doctor bills. Beginning around 1983, managed care emerged as a market force that grew sharply through 1993. In regions where managed care secured a solid foothold, doctors were forced to compete for patients, putting economic pressure on them to change the way they practice. They now had incentives to consider less-expensive medications, decline to provide services of questionable value, and seek other cost-efficient ways to provide care. And it pitted doctor against doctor to see who could provide a service for less. Supply and demand for doctors now had real meaning, as I discuss in detail in Chapter 2. The advent of managed care fundamentally changed the physician marketplace by sharply reducing doctors' control over their practice and their income.

A number of empirical studies have shown that managed care took hold and grew more rapidly in areas that had an oversupply of doctors.[28] In fact, doctor-to-population ratios are important predictors of managed care establishment and growth. We do not suggest that oversupply was the only impetus behind managed care's spread across the country, but *without oversupply, it would not have happened. Why would doctors discount their fees and give up their autonomy?* Competition for patients is the compelling underlying story about how the U.S. health care system evolved over the past few decades, and why. Many observers have thought of managed care as an alien visitor to the planet. In actuality, its origins are distinctly American. Managed care emerged from—and is an indicator of—an oversupply of doctors in the United States.

Doctor Income Drops

In a properly functioning market, an increase in the income of any profession implies that there is a shortage. In contrast, if income is falling, the market is signaling a surplus.[29] This simple proposition did not apply to physicians before the advent of managed care. In the 1960s and 1970s the typical newly trained doctor would move to wherever he (or, far less often, she) wanted to practice, let people know he was in town, and wait for the patients to line up. Usually, the wait wasn't long. These physicians did not have any constraints or economic worries because the system did not deal with doctors as *economic units*, rather as *social goods*. The payment system was passive; whatever doctors did, they were paid for it. This made for a professionally and economically rewarding life for doctors.

Managed Care Maturity

To compete in the managed care environment, however, physicians had to discount their fees substantially—30 percent on average.[30] The resulting drop in incomes, specialty by specialty, is described in Chapter 3.

By making the market work more efficiently, managed care significantly reduced the rate of increase in health care spending between 1993 and 2001, when health maintenance organization (HMO) growth peaked. HMOs had produced health care of high quality while using fewer doctors. In fact, Jonathan Weiner pointed out that HMOs managed to provide high-quality care with doctor-population ratios of 144 to 176 per 100,000. This contrasts sharply with our nation's current ratio: about 229 doctors per 100,000 in 2004.[31]

The period of managed care's maturity brought about another phenomenon that is central to this book. Prior to the market shift introduced by managed care, there had not been any rigorous criteria for determining the right number of doctors for a given population. The United States either had more or fewer doctors per capita than some other country, state, region, or health plan. Therefore, all decisions were made in a relative sense because the demand for doctors was unrelated to the supply. Managed care made it possible, for the first time, to apply market measures—as I will discuss in Chapter 6—to see where the country is now and where we are heading.

Redistribution of Doctor Supply

Because the managed care market is sensitive to demand, it was instrumental in altering the distribution. This is set out in Chapter 4. Market factors also led to the rapid growth in the use of physician assistants and nurse practitioners to effectively increase the size and accessibility of the medical workforce. These professionals perform some two-thirds of the services traditionally provided only by physicians.[32] As I discuss in Chapter 5, they must be included in assessing the market for doctors.

Managed Care Backlash and Decline

Managed care growth reached a peak around 2000, after which it began a gradual decline. The turning point was precipitated by both a physician and consumer backlash, as I discuss in Chapter 2; however it may also reflect the exhaustion of managed care's ability to reduce prices. Nevertheless, managed care has remained a fundamental ingredient of the health care system, and the market signals that it engendered are still at work today.

Where Are We Headed?

To show how these milestones affected the physician supply, we consider them as an overlay to the configuration we call the "Supply Cycle of Doctors," shown in Figure 1.3. This simplified and stylized depiction is, in part, historical because its momentum is propelled by the events I have discussed.

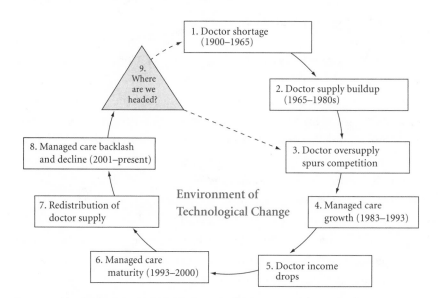

Figure 1.3. The supply cycle of doctors

But it's not *only* historical, because the underlying dynamics are always in play. They will continue to shape the physician supply according to environmental factors that emerge over the coming decades, including shifts in the health care system—especially those driven by new technology—and major changes in society and the economy as a whole. Each step in the supply cycle is based on the data and analysis that I present in the chapters that follow.

ABOUT THIS BOOK

This is a data-driven book. It is grounded in the most recently available data about the health care workforce from a wide variety of sources. Each chapter in Part I drills down into the economic, market, and policy issues relevant to the doctor supply cycle. Several chapters include a close-up view of California, where the supply-cycle dynamics have played out in a particularly dramatic way. Also, a chapter is devoted to international supply-and-demand factors, because health care must increasingly be considered a part of the global economy. However, the emphasis is on the national picture in the United States.

Although the book comes out of an economics perspective, it is not intended to be an academic discussion. The data are interpreted in a way that is intended to be meaningful to health care professionals, medical academics, regulators, health policy professionals, and the public. The book's purpose is to inform the policy debate by bringing a deep understanding of the problems of a health care system that is badly in need of repair. Concerns about access, cost, and quality have become urgent during the past two decades. Reforms that will affect the availability of health insurance coverage are being hotly debated at the federal level and by the states. Such changes are obviously important. But without systemic improvements in the delivery of services, all of these reforms will be unsuccessful; they will simply lead to more frustration for patients, health care professionals, and policymakers alike.

Previous efforts to analyze and fix endemic workforce misalignments have been flawed in their logic and have often exacerbated the problems. This book discusses those initiatives and brings new clarity to the economic forces and market signals that drive health care and its immense workforce, including doctors. It takes into account the enormous complexities of health care delivery and tries to sort out the essential features that need to be changed.

The book's premise is that effective reform must *start* by looking at the delivery side—at the doctors and other health care workers who make it all happen. This is because an efficient, cost-effective, high-quality health care system depends fundamentally on having the right number of doctors, of the right specialty, in the right locations. A corollary to this statement is that the health care delivery workforce *as a whole* must be taken into account. Physicians are truly the engine of medical care, but they make up only a small fraction of caregivers. Their responsibilities are increasingly being shared with other highly skilled workers, in particular nurse practitioners and physician assistants.

Part I concludes with a discussion of the various ways that health economists and others think about the "right" supply of doctors. There is little agreement on which perspective is closest to the mark—or in fact what the mark should be. Nevertheless, I believe that economic factors—in an environment of rapid technological advances—can suggest the direction of the supply cycle over the next five and ten years.

To bring a rich variety of perspectives to this puzzle, I talked with twenty-seven leading figures in the fields of health economics, health policy, and academic medicine. These extraordinary conversations about the health care workforce make up Part II of this book.

Then, in "A Final Word," I leave readers with some observations and reflections on how to improve health care in the United States, and how the role of doctors is likely to be transformed in the coming years. These insights are derived from both the research and analysis spelled out in Part I and the far-ranging discussions in Part II.

In the end, this book is intended to help policymakers and other health care leaders better visualize the economic framework that underlies health care delivery. It provides a multidimensional view of institutional functioning—how health care systems actually operate. This is essential to addressing the fundamental question: How can we significantly improve the efficiency, cost-effectiveness, and quality of health care for Americans? A key part of that process will be determining the "right" supply of doctors, and how best to achieve that.

MANAGED CARE

REDISTRIBUTES MARKET POWER

While his patient was wheeled to recovery, the surgeon stopped by the waiting room to update the patient's anxious family. "Well, I removed 70 percent of the tumor," the surgeon explained. "Why not the whole thing?" they asked. The doctor replied, "The managed care company was only willing to pay 70 percent of my fee."

We have all chuckled at some version of this old story. But for physicians who experienced the transition into the managed-care-controlled marketplace, the sting was real. Before managed care, doctors billed for all their services. More services—consultations, tests, procedures—meant more income. For the most part, patients and third-party payers (both public and private insurers) paid the bill with little resistance. Doctors who maximized their delivery of services in such an environment were behaving rationally, although the outcome was somewhat perverse in terms of unnecessary cost and sometimes questionable quality. This is a phenomenon that economists labeled as moral hazard.[1]

To understand the notion of moral hazard, we'll go back to the culinary world once more. It's the department head's birthday, and the whole staff takes him to dinner at a local restaurant. Because the bill will be evenly shared, the diners have an economic incentive to order the more expensive dishes so that their meal will be subsidized by others. A great opportunity to go for the Surf 'n Turf! Asking for individual checks changes this incentive and eliminates the moral hazard. Moral hazard (unrelated to ethical concerns) occurs when consumers do not bear the full economic consequences of their decision.

The incentives that were applied under managed care were intended to diminish the moral hazard that encouraged excessive services in the fee-for-service environment and resulted in fast-increasing costs for everyone. Managed care encouraged—some would say forced—doctors to practice in a health care marketplace over which they wielded less control than they had become accustomed to. In fact, they saw their professional autonomy, their income, and their economic power greatly reduced. Market power shifted to payers and away from doctors.

Why did this happen? The rapid increase in the ratio of doctors to population tells part of the answer. From 1960 to 1983 the doctor-to-100,000-population ratio increased from 144 to 178, which is an increase of 23 percent.[2] Even with new health care technologies and a growing population pushing up the demand for services, there were not enough patients to go around. Doctors were increasingly obliged to compete for them.

This was a big change for physicians. Before managed care became established, doctors could create demand for their services—called supplier-induced demand.[3] Victor Fuchs, in his landmark analysis of this phenomenon, found that having more surgeons correlates not only with more operations but with higher average cost.[4] Patients with insurance paid very little for physician services, so for decades doctors had the power to manipulate markets.[5] To maintain their incomes, doctors could simply perform more services or provide a more expensive package of care. High spending on health care benefited both physicians and patients, while others paid the bills—as would be the case when the restaurant bill is split among all those at the dinner.

The broken health care market made it impossible to use economic signals, such as changes in the price of care or the income of doctors, to assess the oversupply or undersupply of physicians. Assessments of the shortage or surplus of doctors were based on estimates of the "need" and the availability of doctors to meet it. Need was sometimes defined as whatever physicians believed their patients required; some studies defined need as what epidemiologists believed was needed to treat current or expected patterns of disease. Understandably, health care spending rose dramatically.

Managed care realigned the market by channeling competition for patients into a system that made doctors behave in ways that made health care more cost-effective. Certain aspects of managed care, such as admissions review, second opinions, and selective contracting began to grow.[6] As managed care took hold, these and other demand-reduction techniques were systematized across the industry. Managed care companies now represented demand— because they directed the flow of patients—and physicians represented supply. They brought economic forces to bear on a previously disconnected market in which doctors controlled supply and could influence demand. Payers had a great deal of market power on the demand side, whereas physicians influenced the supply side.

WHAT IS MANAGED CARE?

Managed care is a term that has numerous meanings. What all of them have in common is a contractual relationship between a managed care company and doctors for providing medical services to enrolled members.[7] This contract is more explicit than an old-fashioned insurance contract and therefore may place limits on types of service, providers, or payment amounts. Members pay premiums to the company for a contractually determined range of services to be delivered if and when they are needed. This arrangement creates a market.[8]

There is wide variation in managed care arrangements, but the basic building blocks are physician services and hospital services. A large purchaser, such as an insurance company or a managed care organization, contracts for these services on behalf of its enrollees. In a submarket, large employers typically contract with several managed care companies in order to give their employees a choice of prices and range of services.

There are several other types of managed care arrangements. Independent practice associations (IPAs) restrict insured patients to a defined set of providers, which may be scattered across a region. Preferred provider organizations (PPOs) allow patients to choose any provider, but offer lower deductibles and lower copays to use selected providers within the PPO network; PPOs also monitor the care their network doctors provide. Point-of-service organizations (POSs) allow patients to choose any provider, offering no-deductible and minimal copayment incentives to use select providers while imposing large deductibles and copayments on patients who go outside the network.[9]

By far the best-known type of managed care arrangement is the health maintenance organization (HMO), in which the health insurance plan and the medical staff are fully integrated. HMOs assign doctors to patients, and these doctors have a contractual arrangement with the HMO. Patients who enroll in HMOs might go to hospitals run by the organization. HMOs constitute the oldest and the largest component of strictly capitated insurance plans available today. Under a capitation payment system, the doctor receives a set payment per enrollee, which is intended to cover both the doctor's salary and any costs associated with treating patients. If spending exceeds the capitation rate, the doctor experiences a loss, whereas spending less creates a surplus.

Although all types of managed care organizations have become important in the economy, HMOs were most widespread during the managed care era, and there is much better data on HMOs than on other forms of managed care, as we will see.

DOCTORS AND THE ECONOMICS OF MANAGED CARE

From an economist's perspective, all managed care plans have a few things in common. They require doctors who want to perform expensive services to seek authorization or to follow an agreed-upon protocol. As a result, some services and procedures are not performed, and surpluses or profit margins can be increased.

Managed care, many thought, had the ability to control supplier-induced demand; increased spending on excess or unnecessary services per patient was discouraged because capitation rates were fixed.[10] For instance, HMOs caused a shift from inpatient care to the less expensive outpatient care.[11] Thus managed care reduced physicians' professional autonomy and shifted market power to the managed care plan.

By forcing doctors to swallow the cost of patient care, capitation allowed managed care plans to shift financial risk from the managed care firm to the doctors. It is this risk that creates the incentive for doctors to limit the services, prescriptions, and procedures they provide. In this way, managed care put the risk on the supply side of the market and ameliorated the moral hazard of excess care that dogged the fee-for-service landscape.[12] Hospitals, too, have responded to the incentives of managed care by reducing inpatient care.[13]

Some managed care contracts offered physicians bonuses for keeping hospital admissions down or for saving money in other ways. Physicians began reducing admissions by using more outpatient care and by making sure the patient really needed hospital care before being admitted. For example, an HMO might offer physician groups $10 million to reduce their admissions rate from 30 percent to 25 percent. Managed care organizations figured out that if they saved $20 million by changing physician behavior and gave physicians $10 million, they were still ahead. Not surprisingly, there have been lawsuits about whether or not such arrangements should be allowed.[14] Many people believed these incentives shifted the spectrum of medical services toward the provision of too little care—another form of moral hazard.

Most important, physicians who wanted access to patients through the managed care organizations had to discount their fees, often significantly. On average, managed care companies received 30 percent fee discounts from physicians.[15] Like the fictional surgeon in our opening story, doctors only collected 70 percent of their usual fees.

In addition, managed care organizations forced doctors to play by their rules and have often been quick to expel those who have not cooperated. In 1996, for example, 6 percent of doctors were dropped involuntarily from a managed care plan and 13 percent were denied a contract.[16] In addition, managed care organizations required doctors to give up their autonomy. Physicians in managed care arrangements have to ask someone else—frequently someone with less technical expertise—for permission to perform certain patient care activities.

So managed care arrangements altered two things that physicians hold dear—professional autonomy and earning power. This is a high price to pay and one that doctors did not easily accept. However, the market can be powerful, especially in an era when many believed there was a health care cost crisis.

Managed care did reduce health care costs. It happened for the most part because doctors reduced their fees, but there is scant evidence that the level of care changed. Some high-priced surgical care was avoided because of second opinions. Hospital admissions declined significantly, as did the length of stay. The Kaiser Permanente system, an integrated HMO, has always had lower-than-average hospital costs for these reasons.[17]

MANAGED CARE AND THE PHYSICIAN SURPLUS

Data suggest 1983 as the beginning of the managed care era. At that time, insurance plans were seeking to restrain the fast rise in health care costs through management techniques, such as requiring patients to obtain second opinions before allowing expensive surgeries.[18] But the crucial factor that drove the growth of managed care was excess capacity in the supply of physicians. Figure 2.1 shows that there was a turnaround in both HMO enrollment and physician supply growth in 1999.[19] Doctors needed to compete for patients.

In fact, without an oversupply of doctors, managed care would not likely have grown. If there were enough patient resources to go around, doctors would not have played the managed care game. At the microeconomic level, a number of studies suggest that the oversupply of physicians is a key predictor of the growth of managed care.[20]

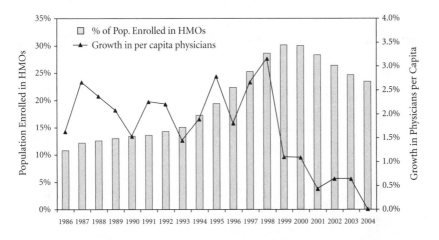

Figure 2.1. HMO enrollment versus growth in supply of physicians per 100,000 population

NOTE: The year 1988 was interpolated.

SOURCES: Data on HMO enrollment from Health and Aging Chartbook, 1993 to 2004. Data on number of physicians from *Physician Characteristics and Distribution in the United States*, American Medical Association, 1997–1998, 1999, 2000, 2001–2002, 2003, and 2005 editions.

MANAGED CARE GROWTH AND MATURITY

HMO penetration grew steadily between 1983 and 1993, from approximately 6 percent to 15 percent of the market. In 1983, physicians reported that 5 percent of their patient contacts involved preferred provider organization (PPO) coverage. Within two years, that fraction had jumped to about 25 percent.[21] By 1993, over 70 percent of all Americans with health insurance were enrolled in some form of managed care plan.[22] As of 1985, approximately 28 percent of the physician population had a contract with a PPO, and this number tripled to 85 percent within ten years.[23] Another way of looking at managed care penetration is the number of practices that had at least one managed care contract. This also started at 28 percent in 1985, but rose to 90 percent in 1997.[24] At the same time, the portion of revenues from Medicaid programs grew. By the late 1990s, doctors were working similar hours but were getting more of their money from managed care and Medicaid.

Because the managed care portion of the market was still relatively small before 1993, it had little effect on physician incomes, staffing, or health care expenditures. It became a major market force between 1993 and 2000 when HMO enrollment grew from 15 percent of the market to 30 percent. In its

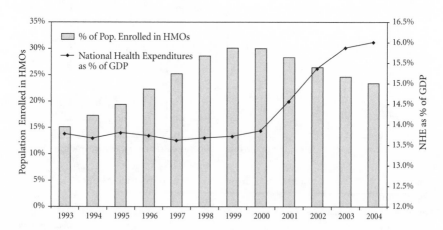

Figure 2.2. HMO enrollment versus national health expenditures as a percentage of GDP, 1993–2004

SOURCES: *National Health Expenditures, 2004*, from Centers for Medicare & Medicaid Services, U.S. Department of Health and Human Services; *Health and Aging Chartbook*, Hyattsville, Maryland: National Center for Health Statistics, 1994, 1999, 2003, 2004, and 2005.

peak years, managed care actually accounted for more of the market than is shown in Figure 2.2; it was probably closer to 50 percent because many PPOs and similar arrangements were also present at that time.

By the early 1990s, managed care's cost-cutting effects had begun to exert a powerful influence on the health care market. This resulted in significant reductions in physician incomes while the number of physician services stayed relatively constant. Lower incomes were driven primarily by a reduction in fees.[25]

Managed care's HMO penetration hit its high point around the year 2000, reaching 30 percent of the market. Penetration has been decreasing slightly every year since; HMOs make up about 25 percent of the market today.

THE IMPACT OF MANAGED CARE ON EXPENDITURES

Managed care helped to slow the growth of health care expenditures. As HMO enrollment increased between 1993 and 2000, health care spending as a percentage of gross domestic product (GDP) stabilized and decreased somewhat. As managed care enrollment fell between 2000 and 2004, expenditures began a strong upward trajectory (see Figure 2.2). This illustrates an important concept: the growth of managed care and the share of GDP devoted to health care spending moved in opposite directions.[26] As managed care grew, health care spending declined, and as managed care declined, health care expenditures rose.[27] The simple correlation between the growth in HMO enrollment and the share of national health expenditures as a percentage of GDP is 0.77.[28]

The managed care market clearly slowed the rate of increase in health care spending, but this wasn't the only cause. Prospective payment in hospitals by Medicare and later on by other payers was an important cost control factor. Prospective payment is a fixed payment for each hospital admission. A federal commission was established to set the fees that doctors received from Medicare. This type of control is akin to price controls imposed by Richard Nixon in the 1970s.[29] The Medicare commission still sets doctors' fees; prospective payment set a payment per admission to the hospital, which varied by the type of admission—essentially a form of capitation.[30]

After managed care was established, the predominant payment mode became capitation and discounted fee for service. Under managed care, financing and delivery of care are integrated. In this environment, physicians had a strong incentive to organize themselves to produce services that competed on price—something they did not have to do in the pre-managed-care world.

THE MANAGED CARE BACKLASH

What caused managed care to peak around 2000 and decline after that? Several things. Doctors started fighting back, and patients decided they wanted an expanded choice of doctors and services and were willing to pay for it. In addition, managed care may have gone as far as it could go in curtailing the medical system; it lowered payments to a point beyond which doctors would not accept further reductions.[31] A backlash was fueled by lawsuits against managed care companies as well as by new government regulations such as the law ending so-called "drive-through deliveries" and guaranteeing postpartum mothers three days in the hospital.[32]

By the time the popular 1997 movie *As Good As It Gets* came out—pitting an asthmatic child and his single mom against a callous health care system dominated by managed care—the public was receptive to its compelling message. Physicians were also becoming frustrated and angry about their loss of autonomy and income under managed care. They began claiming that managed care caused deterioration in the quality of care, a notion that was supported by very few studies.[33]

Another signal of the physician backlash against managed care was the emergence of interest in physician unions as a countervailing power in the marketplace. Doctors understood that they had lost market power. A small fraction of doctors were already involved in unions—state-employed physicians, for example—but the majority were self-employed and did not have any inclination to join a union prior to the growth of managed care. Doctors could not unionize because antitrust laws forbade them to set prices or collude in any way. The Campbell Bill attempted to recalibrate the market, making it legal for self-employed doctors to organize into unions.[34] Although the bill was not successful, doctors who would never have thought about unionizing began discussing it.

In 1999, the American Medical Association (AMA) asked a committee to look into forming a large-scale union.[35] At first, many doctors were viscerally opposed; the committee was famously booed off the stage. But eventually, the AMA did form a union, the Physicians for Responsible Negotiation (PRN).

This was designed to be a professional union, similar to those for university professors and airline pilots. Although it does not sanction strikes, it does allow for the possibility of a slowdown. The union touts its interest in quality, but it serves principally as a consolidated voice for doctors.

Many physicians declined to join the call for unions, but instead joined larger medical groups, which acted as "quasi unions" to negotiate wages and recapture some of doctors' lost autonomy.[36] Doctors began negotiating with managed care organizations through their medical groups to collectively bargain for better wages, benefits, and lifestyles. In fact, Casalino and colleagues found that gaining negotiation leverage with health insurance plans was the most frequently cited benefit of joining a physician organization; the top reasons cited for joining a group practice were lifestyle and income, the same rationale that induces people to join unions.[37] Furthermore, doctors may have achieved some economies of scale in delivering medical services by forming larger groups.[38]

Lawsuits, unions, and the reorganization of physician groups gave physicians the power they needed to fight back against the changes imposed by managed care firms. These mechanisms inevitably played a role in the eventual slowdown of managed care.

CONCLUSIONS

There is strong empirical support for the notion that the oversupply of doctors was a major factor in the rise of managed care. The rapid growth in the supply of doctors per capita was a necessary condition for managed care to make the market more efficient. Doctors now needed to compete for patients. The impact of managed care on doctors was twofold. It took away their autonomy and resulted in the lowering of their fees. Overall growth in health care expenditures as a percentage of GDP slowed as well—a trend that continued until the managed care backlash.

The functioning market created by managed care has enabled the use of market signals—such as physician incomes—to assess shortages and surpluses of doctors. For example, rapidly rising physician incomes could suggest a doctor shortage. By taking market power away from the doctors, managed care made shortages into an observable, measurable phenomenon. The next chapter examines the income of doctors and the resulting market signals.

3

PHYSICIAN INCOMES:

FOLLOWING THE MONEY

A doctor came home from hospital rounds one day to discover that a leaky pipe was flooding his house. He made an urgent call to a plumber, who fixed the leak in two hours and presented a bill for $500. "Are you kidding?" sputtered the doctor. "I don't even charge that much!" The plumber replied, "Well when I was a doctor, I didn't either."

As we have seen, managed care altered the lay of the land for the finance of medical practice. Under capitation and discounted fee-for-service agreements, doctors had strong incentives to be cost-effective in their delivery of health care services. What had been a broken market gained discipline as doctors were forced to negotiate with managed care organizations and insurance companies. The result was a functioning market. How did the presence of this market affect doctors? This chapter takes a look.

HOW MEDICAL PRACTICE HAS CHANGED
AND STAYED THE SAME

To put these changes in context, let's look at the working lives of physicians over the 1983–2001 period. The number of weeks they worked each year, the hours they devoted to nonpatient care, the length of office visits, and the number of patients they saw—all remained relatively unchanged. Here is a snapshot of the working life of doctors during this period:

- Doctor visits averaged about twenty-eight minutes per patient between 1983 and 2001. This is true of both male and female doctors.

- The average number of hours worked per week remained virtually unchanged at 57.8 throughout the period. Though female doctors did work approximately 10 percent fewer hours per week than did male doctors (58.6 hours for men on average versus 52.5 hours for women), these numbers did not change between 1983 and 2001.
- The average number of hours doctors devoted to patient care remained practically constant at 52 hours per week. Also constant since 1983 were the number of hours doctors devoted to nonpatient care (5.5 hours per week) and the number of weeks they worked per year (47.2 weeks).[1]

However, a few things did change between 1983 and 2001. All specialties experienced an upward trend in board certification.[2] In 1983, approximately 65.7 percent of physicians were board certified, but by 2001, the proportion had increased to 81.5 percent. General or family practice, internal medicine, pediatrics, psychiatry, and anesthesiology experienced the biggest growths in certification. General practitioners started at 46 percent and ballooned to 71 percent. Internal medicine started at 67 percent and increased to 87 percent.

Also during this time frame, female doctors caught up to males with regard to board certification. In 1983, roughly two-thirds of the male doctor population was board certified, but only half of female doctors were; by 2001, some 82 percent of male doctors were board certified compared to 80 percent of female doctors.

The increase in size of medical group practices was another significant trend. In 1983, the average doctor practiced in a group of three. By 1993, the average practice size was 3.8 doctors, and by 2001, it was 4.7—an increase of 56.7 percent between 1983 and 2001. Two hospital-based specialties experienced especially dramatic increases in the average number of doctors per practice. Radiologist practices grew from 5.6 to 7.6 doctors, and anesthesiologist groups went from an average of 4.7 to 6.2 members.

Income Changes

An analysis of physician incomes over time tells an interesting story. To see how physician incomes have changed, it is useful to look at trends across two contiguous periods in the evolution of managed care: the beginning and gradual growth era (1983–1993), and the maturity and decline period (1993–2000). The dates correlate with the rapid takeoff of managed care in 1993.[3]

The income trajectories for all physicians—as well as for hospital-based and nonhospital-based specialists—are displayed in Figure 3.1. Physicians as a whole enjoyed a steady rise in income during the period when managed care was just beginning to pick up traction; earnings peaked at $220,000 in 1993 and saw a slight decline afterward. In that same year, incomes for hospital-based doctors topped out at $300,000, while earnings of practice-based doctors peaked at $170,000. After 1993, hospital-based doctors experienced a sizable decline in their incomes, whereas practice-based specialists did not, even though their income was flat in real terms (adjusted for inflation).

In sum, the inflation-adjusted income of doctors peaked in 1993, matching the takeoff of managed care. If wages are considered as market signals, the decline in the income of hospital-based doctors suggests that there was a surplus of those doctors at that time, and the slight rise in the income of practice-based doctors suggests that there was a small shortage.

The decline in U.S. doctor income by specialty is further delineated in Figure 3.2. Again, the analysis focuses on two periods: the decade before the income peak in 1993—as managed care entered its maturity phase—and the nine years afterward. Using real income deflated for the cost of living, I found that the earnings of doctors increased an annual average of 5.1 percent from

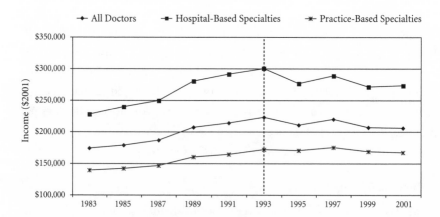

Figure 3.1. Average physician net income by specialty grouping, 1983–2001

NOTE: Hospital-based specialties include pathology, radiology, surgery, and anesthesiology. Practice-based specialties include gp / fp, internal medicine, psychiatry, ob / gyn, and pediatrics. The "other" specialty category has been excluded from these two groupings, but has been included in the "all doctors" average.

SOURCE: AMA Socioeconomic Monitoring System Data.

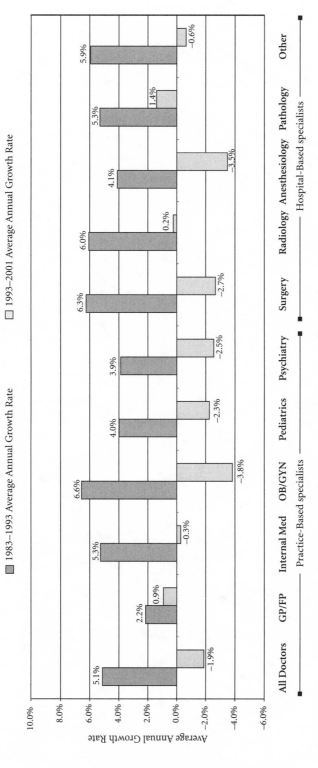

Figure 3.2. Average annual growth in real physician net income ($2001), 1983–1993 versus 1993–2001

SOURCE: Analysis of AMA Socioeconomic Monitoring System data, 1983, 1985, 1987, 1989, 1991, 1993, 1995, 1997, 1999, and 2001.

Table 3.1. Physician incomes and growth rates by specialty

	Incomes in $2006 Dollars							Growth Rates (percentage)		
	1983	1993	2001	2002–2003	2003–2004	2004–2005	2005–2006	1983–1993	1993–2001	1983–2001
All Professions*	40,901	47,728	62,138	N/A	N/A	N/A	N/A	1.6	3.4	2.4
All Doctors	196,845	252,195	233,041	N/A	N/A	N/A	N/A	2.5	-1.0	0.9
Radiology	268,553	357,248	351,284	344,876	356,724	365,811	351,000	2.9	-0.2	1.5
Anesthesiology	265,708	320,814	277,206	315,502	318,504	312,227	306,000	1.9	-1.8	0.2
Surgery	258,913	347,796	311,189	263,281	263,296	262,765	272,000	3.0	-1.4	1.0
OB/GYN	226,200	306,349	257,099	257,841	256,926	254,522	234,000	3.1	-2.2	0.7
Pathology	214,578	269,627	279,248	NA	NA	NA	NA	2.3	0.4	1.5
Internal Medicine	175,031	224,972	222,069	NA	NA	NA	NA	2.5	-0.2	1.3
Psychiatry	152,689	183,452	165,053	176,246	174,115	181,360	174,000	1.9	-1.3	0.4
GP/FP	143,899	158,867	163,924	158,839	155,005	154,568	145,000	1.0	0.4	0.7
Pediatrics	142,032	171,936	156,116	NA	NA	NA	NA	1.9	-1.2	0.5
Other	178,248	236,766	226,708	NA	NA	NA	NA	2.9	-0.5	1.4

NOTES: *From BLS average weekly hours (EES00500040) times average wage per hour (EES00500049) times 52.

1983 to 1993. Then, from 1993 to 2001, income fell an average of 1.9 percent annually. Of all specialties, ob/gyns had the largest increase in the pre-1993 period (6.6 percent annually), followed by surgeons (6.3 percent), and radiologists (6.0 percent). General practitioners and family physicians had a very small increase before 1993 (2.2 percent per year) and an increase of just 0.9 percent per year after 1993.

In the mature managed care period—after 1993—ob/gyns and anesthesiologists experienced a dramatic decrease in income of 3.8 percent and 3.5 percent, respectively. Declines were seen in the incomes of specialists in pediatrics, psychiatry, and surgery. Internists saw almost no change in their real income—a 0.3 percent decline (Table 3.1).

Figure 3.1 shows these changes in terms of dollars. The analysis suggests that, in the managed care maturity period, 1993–2001, the demand and supply of physicians as a whole were roughly in balance. However, there were significant differences by specialty.

Differences by Specialty

A look at the income of generalists and various types of specialists over time tells an equally interesting story within the overall pattern. Two specialties that did better on average before the managed care maturity period were ob/gyn and surgery, which experienced average annual income increases of over 6 percent (as compared to 5.1 percent for doctors as a group). In the post-managed-care period, the income for these two specialties fell an annual average of 3.3 percent per year. Contrast this with the 1.9 percent decline for doctors overall.

In general, the highest-paid doctors were the hardest hit by the earnings decline. The specialties that experienced greater-than-average income decline were ob/gyn, pediatrics, psychiatry, surgery, and anesthesiology, which indicates that these specialties were in oversupply before 1993. Although most specialties fared poorly under managed care, general practice and family practice physicians were not hit as hard.

To further understand these income changes, I looked at the income of doctors from 1983 to 2001 and applied statistical controls[4] for the following factors: age of the doctor, gender, number of years in practice after medical school, specialty, board certification, and whether or not trained in the United States.[5] After taking all these factors into account, I found a very similar result—that the average annual income of doctors increased 5 percent per year in the decade before 1993, and declined 1.4 percent annually afterward. This analysis also indicated that some of the income decline was due to factors that were controlled for (such as changes in specialty mix or gender balance), but almost 80 percent was not. Thus 80 percent of the decline likely could be attributed to market forces.

A third way in which the impact of managed care on the market for doctors can be measured is through its effect on medical students' choice of specialties when they apply to residency programs (see Figure 3.3). Although the incomes of primary care specialists—defined as general and family practitioners, internists, and pediatricians—went up between 1993 and 2001, the incomes of nonprimary care specialists declined. The number of applicants to primary care residency positions went up after 1993, and the number of applicants for nonprimary care residencies was essentially flat until 1999, with a slight uptick

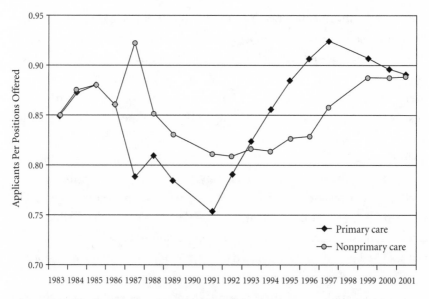

Figure 3.3. Demand for residency positions: Primary and nonprimary care specialties, 1983–2001

NOTE: Data points for 1989 and 1994 are interpolated.

DATA SOURCES: "Results for the Nation Resident Matching Program," for years 1983–2001 from *Academic Medicine*.

after that. I surmised that the market produced a drop in demand for specialties whose income had declined, and an upswing in demand for specialties whose income rose—a clear market signal.

So I observed that, not surprisingly, incomes do influence the choice of residency positions.[6] Over time, teaching hospitals also adjust their supply of residency positions to meet the demands of the market.

Winners and Losers

The disparity in incomes of doctors mirrors the narrative set out in the introduction to this volume in which restaurant popularity reveals quality differences but does not offer insights into overall supply. Medicine, of course, provides a more compelling framework: if you need a certain doctor, and you believe your health or your life depends on it, you may not care how much it costs.[7] Like high-profile restaurants, very prominent doctors are less controlled by managed care than are other doctors, and can therefore charge more.

In 1983, some 28 percent of all doctors attained incomes of $400,000, but by 2001, this proportion had declined to 17 percent, adjusted for inflation. The 19 percent of doctors earning $100,000 or less in 1983 likewise decreased to 11 percent by 2001. However, as we take a closer look at the impact of managed care's growing influence during the 1990s, we find that higher earners experienced different effects than lower earners. Table 3.2 summarizes the changes that have occurred from 1983 to 2001 for doctors earning less than $100,000 and those earning $400,000 or over.

Table 3.2. Analysis of top and bottom earners, 1983 versus 2001 ($2001)

	Under $100,000			$400,000 and Over		
	1983	2001	Difference	1983	2001	Difference
Avg. Yearly Income	$66,671	$65,435	−$1,235	$522,706	$537,229	$14,523
Avg. Hours Worked (total)	53.1	50.2	−2.9	58.8	58.2	−0.6
Avg. Weeks Worked	45.5	46.8	1.4	45.4	47.0	1.6

SOURCE: AMA Socioeconomic Monitoring System data, 1983, 1985, 1987, 1989, 1991, 1993, 1995, 1997, 1999, and 2001.

In 2001 dollars, those at the top experienced a 3 percent increase in their annual salary on average—from $522,706 in 1983 to $537,229 in 2001—whereas those at the bottom had a 2 percent decline—from $66,671 in 1983 to $65,435. In other words, the $456,035 earnings differential in 1983 between top and bottom earners increased to $471,793 by 2001. A portion of the gap can be explained by the hours-worked factor. The physicians at the bottom worked almost three hours fewer than before (about 6 percent less), while those at the top continued to work about the same number of hours. However, the average hourly income for top earners increased by 80 percent, from $186 to $335, compared with only 54 percent for doctors earning less than $100,000, from about $31 to $48. What we find is that fewer doctors are taking a bigger slice of the pie.

Not surprisingly, the specialty with the largest representation in the top group is surgery, at 35.3 percent; the one most represented in the bottom group is general practice and family practice at 25.4 percent. In terms of age, those between 42 and 61 make up greater percentages of the top 20 percent than they do the bottom 20 percent. Physicians at the top are more likely to be practice owners or part owners, to provide Medicare services, to not be employed by hospitals, and to not provide Medicaid services. They earn less income from managed care: 39.3 percent of the top group's income comes from managed care, whereas 46.7 percent of the bottom group's revenue comes from that source.[8]

The fact that higher-income doctors take fewer managed care patients is no coincidence. It suggests that doctors with market power want to avoid bossy managed care firms. Much as high-end restaurants can be choosy about which neighborhoods to locate in, high-end doctors can be discerning about which insurance types to accept.

Differences by Age

The distribution of wages across a doctor's lifetime depends on two main factors: the value added from work experience and the depreciation of the doctor's medical education as new techniques replace those he or she learned in medical school. For the first ten years out of residency, the experience factor plays the biggest role. As a result, doctors between the ages of forty-two and fifty-one earn about 16 percent more on average than those below forty-two. However, after the age of fifty-one, the depreciation of the medical education slows down salary growth. For instance, doctors between fifty-two and sixty-one earn less than 1 percent more than those in the forty-two to fifty-one age bracket. Doctors over sixty-two actually earn less on average than new doctors out of residency. This happens because the older doctors went to medical school at a time before many treatments and technologies had even been discovered.

Gender Gap

It is useful to examine gender differences in income to see how women physicians have fared under managed care. During the period we are looking at, women became physicians in significantly greater numbers, increasing from 8.5 percent of the physician workforce in 1983 to approximately 21.4 percent in 2001. And this trend has continued. Currently, the number of women in medical school is about half the total,[9] and the number of women in residency is approximately 40 percent.[10] They appear to have reached gender parity in numbers. But what about earnings?

A stark pattern emerges in Table 3.3. In 2001, women represented just 16 percent of all physicians earning $400,000 or above, but 45 percent of those earning less than $100,000. Although women have increasingly become physicians in greater numbers, they are disproportionately represented at the lower end of the income spectrum.

In the evolution of managed care over time, the income of female physicians follows a pattern similar to that of male physicians, although the dollar amounts are significantly lower. About 15 percent of the gender differential is due to hours worked. Women physicians worked 10.6 percent fewer hours than men, and earned 33 percent less on average.[11] After controlling for specialty,

Table 3.3. Mean annual net income for male and female physicians ($2006)

	1983	1993	2001
All Doctors	$196,845	$252,195	$233,041
Men	$203,066	$267,798	$252,673
Women	$128,352	$164,331	$158,660

SOURCE: AMA Socioeconomic Monitoring System data, 1983, 1985, 1987, 1989, 1991, 1993, 1995, 1997, 1999, and 2001.

number of years in practice, whether trained in the United States, and hours and weeks worked, there remains a 20 percent differential in the earnings of women compared to men that cannot be explained by these factors. In 2001, doctors as a group averaged $233 thousand in income; males earned $253 thousand, while females made $159 thousand—about 37 percent less.

Moreover, the gap between male and female physician incomes increased from 19.5 percent before managed care to 21.2 percent in the post-managed-care period, suggesting that the income gap was not reduced by managed care.

HOW PHYSICIANS ARE PAID

We can see that market dynamics expressed as income appear to work well in reducing shortages and surpluses. However, many believe as I do that it is even more important to look at *how* we pay physicians, rather than simply how *much* we pay them. The traditional methods are salary, fee-for-service (piece rate), capitation, and combinations of these. More recently, there has been substantial literature about the payment of bonuses to achieve certain results—usually quality, outcomes, or cost-savings indicators. This concept, referred to as pay for performance (P4P), is generally understood as aligning the payment system for a given group of providers so that better performance is rewarded with a higher reimbursement rate.[12]

Although the idea is appealing, there are a number of measurement issues that must be overcome with this type of payment scheme. Not surprisingly, there are various ways of assessing performance, and each has its own set of problems. Simply producing more services could impinge on quality, whereas focusing on quality to the exclusion of quantity would not be practical. Also, there are conflicting opinions about who should receive the reward—the individual doctor, the medical group, or the hospital? Finally, the level of reward necessary to achieve the desired performance is not well understood. Setting the amount of reward too high or the goals too low risks a distortion of the system and unwanted corollary effects. This happened recently in England, resulting in skyrocketing incomes for primary care doctors.[13]

To date, the research shows that the amounts of incentive pay in place in the United States are too low to have a significant impact on physician behavior.[14] Nevertheless, it's quite clear that P4P is going to be with us at least for the foreseeable future. Numerous experiments—hundreds perhaps—are under way throughout the country to develop reliable, measurable P4P mechanisms. I see this as part of a growing national intolerance for financial waste and inattention to quality in the health care system. Medicare recently raised the stakes for hospitals and physicians by refusing to pay hospitals for avoidable errors.[15] This will undoubtedly affect quality for the better as other payers follow Medicare's lead. As has been seen over the past forty years, policy changes that directly or indirectly affect incomes subsequently appear as market signals.

The most cutting-edge research in this area reveals very little evidence that P4P has a significant effect on treatment behaviors.[16] Researchers in this particular study looked at a newly implemented P4P program and found that, for the most part, it followed trends similar to another group who had not used P4P.

In fact, as the authors of a very thorough review of all P4P literature note, almost every academic study of P4P reveals that doctors do not respond much to P4P incentives.[17] These authors take a step back to look at the bigger-picture lessons gleaned from the aggregate of these studies. Most of these interventions have been small scale. They point out that it really isn't worth the doctors' time to pay attention to small interventions. Because doctors receive payment from so many different payers, if one payer pays them to change a specific aspect of their practice, the cost (in effort) of making that change is not worth the marginal payment that a particular provider offers. If P4P is going to have potential, it will probably require many payers to coordinate efforts so that the doctor's behavior is rewarded across the board. Some national nonprofit groups have formed to try to coordinate across payers, and these groups are slowly infiltrating the system.

Because of these coordinating factors, one's understanding is incomplete without a bigger-picture perspective of what's happening on the P4P frontier. Thankfully, there is a very recent study that has looked at the infiltration of P4P in HMOs across the country.[18] Because HMOs respond so powerfully to financial incentives, their behavior can act as an indicator of what will work going forward. As it turns out, in areas with greater emphasis on primary care, HMOs are more likely to use P4P. Without a primary care physician, it is difficult to pin down one party responsible for a patient's treatment. The study also finds that HMOs target P4P efforts at physician groups rather than individual physicians. This spreads some of the risk and also gives doctors a social incentive to comply with quality standards. These broad-scale studies can tell us a great deal about the direction of P4P going forward. We will be wise to heed these lessons.

COST OF TRAINING AND RATE OF RETURN

This chapter has shown that physicians have high income, on average, even though it has fluctuated over time. Why do they make so much? Clearly part of the answer is that they provide services that people value and that society is willing to pay good money for. But that's not the end of the story. The high cost of medical education necessitates high salaries later in life. Otherwise students would not be willing to pay the up-front cost of their own training.

This raises the question, How much does it cost to train a doctor? I did some calculations, and estimate that it costs society about $1 million to train a doctor with four years of medical school and four years of internship and residency (see Appendix A for details). This amount includes instructional costs for medical school and training costs associated with residency. If one were to tack on the other educational resources involved in training a medical student, it would bring the total cost of training a doctor to $1.6 million. The extra $0.6 million includes research costs and other resources that have value to society apart from educating the doctor. For purposes of this book, we refer to the $1 million figure for the cost of training a doctor. In addition to direct training costs, the figures also include the wages the doctor forgoes during the years of training. Economists refer to this as the "opportunity cost,"[19] and it is generally an important part of the costs associated with training. If the opportunity costs were not included, it would cost around $329,000 to train a doctor. Still a lot of money.

But are those costs worth it? The rate of return provides us with one measure of the economic value of the medical training. Much as a stock share has a rate of return on investment, so does education. The return on education accounts for the services that the doctor will provide to people after finishing training. It essentially measures how many services society gets back for each dollar put into medical school and residency programs. Society includes all stakeholders, such as the medical student, the government, private donors, and anyone else who contributes directly or indirectly to the cost of training. Despite the high cost of training, this return is still larger than the general return on education per year of nonmedical schooling, which is 8.5 percent.[20]

Of course, doctors bear only a fraction of the costs of their medical training. They bear about $550,000 of their training costs if one includes their opportunity cost, or the wages they forgo in order to attend school. This is just over half of the total cost of medical education. Because they enjoy higher salaries for the rest of their working lives, their personal return on investment is quite high. There is roughly a 23 percent personal return on investment for specialists and a 19 percent personal return for general practitioners.[21] These figures fall in line with other professional degrees. For instance, a graduate degree in business will bring a 29 percent rate of return, a law degree a 25.4 percent return, and a dental degree a 20.7 percent return.[22] So even though they make high salaries, doctors still have a lower return on education than do lawyers and M.B.A.s! This helps put things into perspective.

CONCLUSIONS

By shifting the market signals for physicians, managed care made it possible to understand the significant changes in income over time and by specialty. These changes signal the shortages and surpluses of physicians. In 1993, the real income of doctors peaked and then declined slightly until 2001, suggesting that the market for physicians was becoming oversupplied. In a managed care system, primary care doctors had their incomes rise while those of most specialties declined. Residents responded to income signals by increasing the demand for primary care residencies and reducing the demand for specialty training. However, this trend ended around 1997, and by 2001, the demand for specialty training was equal to that of primary care.

Following the build-up in both numbers and power of primary care physicians (PCPs) during the early managed care era, the popularity of primary care residencies for American-trained medical students has dropped. Already burdened by educational debt, students know they will earn substantially more as specialists, and residency programs know they will get more valuable services from specialists they train. The marketplace is generally not kind to PCPs, and their income has been dropping steadily.

Nevertheless, many experts continue to emphasize the centrality of the PCP role as an entry point to the health care system and as a trusted coordinator of care for the patient—especially in chronic care.[23] The idea of the "medical home," which has gained a great deal of attention in the past few years, hinges on the central role of primary-care, office-based practice. With the backing of the American Academy of Pediatrics, pilot studies have been under way to test the value of the PCP office as a central hub for records, communication, and coordination of care, especially for chronically ill and disabled children.[24] An important factor in such arrangements is the reimbursement of physicians for their time, as well as for the staffing and electronic information and communication systems necessary for the coordination tasks.

The overarching pressure for cost-efficiency, especially given the burgeoning demand for effective chronic care, is challenging boundaries between primary and specialty care. This pressure is a factor in the emergence of such innovations as P4P, the medical home, and other ways to enhance the value of the doctors—particularly the primary care doctors.

WHO ARE THE DOCTORS,

AND WHERE ARE THEY?

During my second year on the faculty at the University of North Carolina in Chapel Hill, I was asked to think about the following question: What would be the best strategy to increase the number of physicians in the state of North Carolina? One possibility was to build a two-year medical school in East Carolina and have the students transfer to UNC Chapel Hill for their third and fourth years. The other proposed solution was to somehow attract physicians from outside the state.

After a summer spent analyzing this problem, I was called to a deans' meeting to present my findings. I explained that, instead of building a new medical school, it would be much more cost-effective to provide higher salaries to physicians to come into the state, and even to offer housing subsidies and private school tuitions to their children. These measures, I pointed out, would produce 50 to 75 percent more physicians in the next ten years than would any possible build-up at East Carolina or Chapel Hill medical schools. The deans' council thanked me for my rigorous analysis. Then the chairman asked, "Professor Scheffler, do you think the job of being a doctor is a good one?"

I said "Of course. Being a doctor is considered to be a high-status job, and it's highly paid."

"If you think so, Professor Scheffler, why should we give those good jobs to northerners? What would they know about the health problems of people in North Carolina?" And so the panel made a formal recommendation to build a medical school over in East Carolina.

What is the message? It illustrates that physician supply policy cannot be determined from a single perspective because it has important societal, political, health care, and economic ramifications. Often the same policy body that makes decisions about access to health care for a population is also concerned with political and economic considerations. This makes the supply question a lot more complicated. There is no single policy that can be followed.

Of course, there is some merit to the Chapel Hill panel's argument in terms of primary care. It is important for a primary care physician to understand his or her patients—to know where they grew up and be familiar with the culture of the region. But some specialties may be different. If a neurosurgeon has little in common with the patient, it matters less. Neurosurgeons—and most subspecialists—may not need personal relationships with their patients. Their interaction with patients is on a different level than that between primary care doctors and their patients.

The deans' panel also had a point in their conviction that physicians trained in North Carolina would be more likely to stay in the state—and conversely that those Yankees would probably leave once the subsidy ran out. The faculty didn't see why North Carolina should spend taxpayer money on them. In fact, at that time, physicians who attended medical school and residency in the same state were very likely to practice there.[1]

This experience taught me that physician supply and distribution policy is a lot more complex than it first appears. California is currently using this argument as part of a proposal to expand the number of medical schools in the state. The proponents argue that Californians should not have to leave home for medical training, nor should the state depend on importing doctors.[2]

BARRIERS TO OPTIMAL DISTRIBUTION

Conceptually, there may be an optimal distribution of physicians—depending on which of various objectives are desired—but attaining such an "ideal" configuration is an ongoing and difficult effort. In general, society is considered to have a responsibility to provide a doctor for those who need one, but for some communities this challenge can be acute.

A host of questions must be asked and answered over time. What size town has the societal right to have a doctor to provide medical care? Should every community of forty people or more have a doctor? One hundred people? One thousand people? How close should the doctor be? Half an hour away? An hour?

The geographic distribution of physicians is a particular problem in the United States, unlike in the many countries in which doctors are steered to areas of particular need after they graduate from medical school. For example, the United Kingdom has a system that attempts to place doctors paid by the National Health Service in areas of need. American doctors are free to move wherever they would like to practice, within the limits of state licensing.

THREE MEASURES OF DISTRIBUTION

Let's look at three different ways to assess distribution of doctors—spatially, by specialty, and by race or ethnicity.

Spatial distribution refers to how well physicians are distributed throughout a geographic area. For example, if there are many more physicians per hundred thousand people in urban areas than in rural ones, it can be said that physicians are poorly distributed across the locale. *Specialty* distribution refers to specialization in medicine. For example, if a region has a shortage of primary care physicians, but an overabundance of some specialists, it could be said that the distribution of specialties is poor. *Racial or ethnic* distribution refers to how well the ethnic makeup of physicians in a region matches that of the population. For example, if 30 percent of a region's population is Hispanic, but only 15 percent of its physicians are of the same heritage, the racial or ethnic distribution is discordant.

Has managed care improved spatial or geographic distribution of doctors? One way to answer this question is to look at distribution over the period of managed care's growth and maturity. I calculated the coefficient of variation (CV) for the per capita number of doctors for the United States and California, by county, over time. The coefficient measures the "evenness" of the distribution of physicians across a geographical unit by dividing the distribution's standard deviation by the mean. We can see from Figure 4.1 that the CV increased from 1983 to about 1993, and then decreased after 1995. The rise indicates that the distribution of physicians was getting worse, and the subsequent drop means that the distribution was improving.

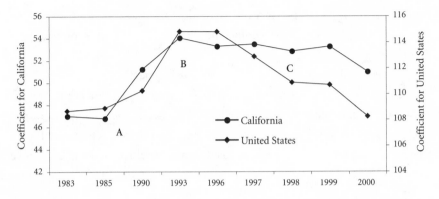

Figure 4.1. Coefficient of variation for physician distribution, California versus the United States

NOTE: Between points A and B, the physician-to-population ratio rose. But after 1993, this ratio fell. The standard deviation of the physician-to-population ratio rose between points A and B, such that it was relatively high by 1993. This indicates a less even distribution of doctors. The standard deviation dropped in the post-1993 period, as the distribution of physicians across geographical areas became more even.

SOURCE: Area Resource File, 2003.

It is interesting to observe that the rise and decline of the CV for the United States and for California followed a very similar pattern. There was a population exodus from urban areas in California and across the United States during these two decades—the coefficient of variation of the population density of California counties steadily dropped from 1983 to 2000.[3] In 1993 physicians began moving away from urban areas, and, as can be seen in Figure 4.1, the CV of physician-population ratio started to decline.[4] More suburban and rural areas experienced the highest growth rate increases in physicians per capita during the 1993–2000 period.[5] Across the United States, the growth in number of physicians after 1993 increasingly gained momentum the further away from urban centers when compared with the growth in physicians before that year. In California, suburban areas in particular experienced the highest increases in the growth rates of physicians per capita after 1993. This pattern mirrored the increase in managed care, with a tipping point at about 1993, as we have seen in Chapter 2. As the managed care market matured, the CV declined, suggesting an improvement in the distribution of physicians.

Therefore, the growth in managed care—not simply the outward migration of doctors—helped to alter the distribution of doctors to population. Though managed care was not the only factor affecting distribution, it clearly was an important one.

The mature managed care market is more sensitive to demand for services than was the market environment of managed care's early growth period. Market forces motivate the demand and supply of health care services toward a balance or equilibrium.[6] High managed care penetration meant that doctors could no longer hang out a shingle and expect patients to come. To get access to patients, doctors had to contract with managed care firms, and those organizations steered them to places where they perceived there was actual need. Whereas specialist physicians generally left areas where managed care penetration was growing the fastest prior to 1993, they began returning to such areas after that year. This geographic movement of physicians in tandem with growth in HMOs suggests that physicians responded to managed care's influence in balancing both the spatial and specialty distribution of doctors.[7] Specialist physicians avoid areas of rising managed care penetration; however, this effect is muted in areas of rising income.

Another way to look at the distribution of physicians is to consider the differences between specialists and nonspecialists. Unlike primary care physicians, specialists often require large population densities to maintain a steady patient pool. Specialists, such as neurosurgeons, only treat a very small portion of the population; if they located in small towns, they would see a handful of people per week and would not be able to maintain a viable practice.[8] Managed care organizations analyze their particular population's needs in order to distribute specialists and nonspecialists in a cost-effective way.

There are many reasons for concern about racial or ethnic discordance. Language barriers can reduce the quality of care, and some treatments may not be appropriate when cultural factors are correctly taken into account.[9] These concerns are most serious for primary care doctors because of their initial and central role in patient care and communication. In the United States, even though fully 14 percent of the population is of Hispanic or Latino origin, only 5 percent of all physicians are, suggesting that Hispanics may encounter more obstacles than individuals of other races or ethnicities when seeking medical care.[10] African-Americans are similarly underrepresented, comprising less than 4 percent of the physician workforce but nearly 13 percent of the population.

In contrast, Caucasian and Asian physicians are overrepresented in comparison with the U.S. population. There are income effects. For example, in areas where Hispanic physicians are underrepresented relative to the Hispanic population, they have higher earnings per hour than non-Hispanic doctors.[111] This result suggests that Hispanic patients place value on being treated by Hispanics. Is it language or culture that accounts for this? It's difficult to say from this result. Language is a strong contender, especially for immigrants. I can imagine that the language issue is key in primary care, but for fields such as surgery, it seems less important because the technical ability of the doctor would likely be the priority, not the ethnic background.

CLOSE-UP ON CALIFORNIA

California, with the largest penetration of HMOs in the country,[12] offers a compelling close-up of distribution issues related to managed care's growth and maturity periods. In this section, we look at a number of measures that illustrate this: ratio of physicians to population, income factors, urban-rural distribution, and racial or ethnic match between doctors and patient populations.

It is interesting to look at the number of physicians in California compared with the rest of the country. Figure 4.2 shows that California had a significantly greater ratio of physicians to population throughout the managed care growth period, but this discrepancy steadily narrowed. In 2001, the last year

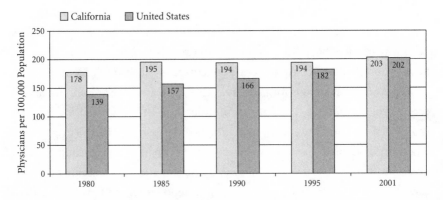

Figure 4.2. Patient care physician-to-population ratio, 1980–2001
SOURCE: Petris Center analysis of the AMA Masterfile.

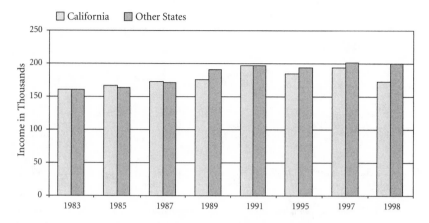

Figure 4.3. Real income of California and U.S. physicians, 1983–1998 ($1998)
SOURCE: Petris Center analysis of AMA Socioeconomic Status Surveys, 1983–1998.

in which figures are available, the ratios were virtually identical. It is true that California had an increase in population that exceeded the rest of the country. To maintain its ratio, California needed to attract doctors and discourage them from emigrating from the state.

Many factors affect migration into and out of California, but income in a state characterized by high living expenses is an important one. Comparing the income of doctors in California with that of doctors in the nation overall from 1983 to 1998, Figure 4.3 indicates that income levels for both were roughly the same in the beginning of this period. In 1989, there was a small dip during which California doctors earned a bit less than in the country as a whole, but by 1991 income levels were the same again. After 1991, California's doctors saw a decline in income, and by 1998 the income discrepancy was significant— about $178,000 for California doctors versus $200,000 for the nation. Doctors found it less economically desirable to locate their practices in California as their incomes fell and living expenses increased. Some practicing doctors left the state, and some graduating doctors decided to practice elsewhere.

These income changes can also be observed through the number of actively practicing specialty doctors in California relative to the rest of the United States (see Figure 4.4). By 2001, as managed care entered its downward trend, there was a ratio of 114 specialists to 100,000 population in California,

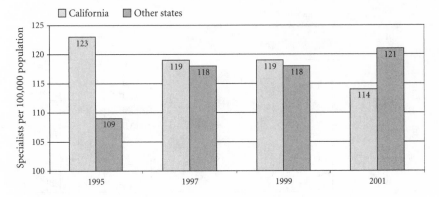

Figure 4.4. Ratios of specialist physicians to population, California and other states, 1995–2001

SOURCE: Petris Center analysis of AMA physician characteristics and distribution reports for select years.

compared with 121 per 100,000 population in other states. Contrast this with 1995 ratios, which showed the reverse relationship. What drove that change was, in part, managed care's impact on income. It was clearly one of the most important factors, but not the only one. Changes in the specialty mix and state payment regulations also played a part.

RACIAL OR ETHNIC MATCH BETWEEN DOCTORS AND POPULATIONS

In California, we also find racial or ethnic maldistribution, using the racial or ethnic composition of the population as a normative benchmark for the diversity of the physician workforce.[13]

Caucasians are overrepresented in the physician population: some 48 percent of all Californians are Caucasian, but fully 65 percent of the state's doctors are. Likewise, Asians are overrepresented in the physician workforce: the population is roughly 12 percent Asian, but 23 percent of the physician population shares that ethnicity. In contrast, African-Americans are underrepresented in the doctor population: about 8 percent of Californians are African-American, but only 4 percent of physicians are. Hispanics have the worst discordance; they make up 32 percent of the population but only 5 percent of the physician workforce.[14]

This racial or ethnic discordance has been found to exist over time and is unlikely to change in the foreseeable future, given the makeup of the current residency pool in California. In fact, the underrepresentation of Hispanic physicians is becoming worse. The overrepresentation of Caucasian physicians is decreasing slightly, but that is primarily driven by the increase in Asian physicians.

Future imbalances will likely be affected by the large discrepancy in incoming medical school students: although Hispanics make up the fastest-growing segment of the California population, Asians constitute the fastest-growing portion of medical school students.

All this suggests that the ethnic disproportion between populations and physicians is a problem in California. But there are at least two mitigating factors. First, language proficiency among physicians may help to moderate communication barriers. Second, minority physicians are more likely to work in underserved areas.[15] Hispanic physicians earn more in areas where the degree of potential racial or ethnic concordance between physicians and patients is lower than the potential demand for such relationships. Language concordance is likely the main reason for this finding.[16]

CONCLUSIONS

There will always be a maldistribution of physicians. The movement of the population happens at a faster pace than the movement of doctors can match. The optimal distribution of doctors from a health point of view is not likely to be the same as that produced by the market. For purposes of health, we may want the distribution of doctors by geography and specialty to meet underlying health needs. It often does, but the functioning of the health care market also means that economic factors are in play. Doctors, like others in society, respond to economic incentives, including income.

Managed care heightened the influence of the market and had a dramatic impact on the distribution of doctors, though money is not the only factor. Doctors are a caring lot, and they want to do the right thing, which some interpret as serving minorities and practicing in underserved areas. Marketplace factors alone do not necessarily provide broad access to health care or distribute doctors equitably across the population. Like the distribution of plates at the dinner party discussed in Chapter 1, the market does not allocate doctors in a socially desirable way; it distributes them where the economic resources are available for them to practice. The market itself does not accomplish social goals, such as adequate access to health care for all. This is why—although it is important to have a properly functioning market for physician services—there is an important role for government and social policy in ensuring equitable access.

5

RESHAPING THE WORKFORCE:

NURSE PRACTITIONERS AND

PHYSICIAN ASSISTANTS

We have all been to the theater, and we know the disappointment of finding out that an understudy will replace the lead performer. We had been looking forward to seeing the star of the show. However, we soon find out that the substitute is very good—an understudy for the lead would have to be quite talented. The performance seems perfectly adequate to us, and we enjoy ourselves, giving little thought to the lack of the headliner.

To a surprising extent, this is similar to the experience of patients when they are served by a nurse practitioner (NP) or a physician assistant (PA), rather than by a doctor. Why is this phenomenon important to our discussion of the doctor supply? There are a number of reasons, as this chapter details. But the main reason to look in depth at the scope of work performed by NPs and PAs is because these frontline health workers perform tasks that physicians would otherwise do. They therefore must be considered in any analysis or forecast of the medical workforce. Their emergence as a strong presence in the workforce grew out of the market reconfiguration produced by managed care. NPs and PAs belong to a category of health services providers sometimes referred to as advanced practice clinicians. Certified nurse practitioners and other providers can be included in this designation. For the purposes of this book I will focus on NPs and PAs.

In a sense, these professionals can be thought of as doctors with a different scope of practice. NPs and PAs can handle 70 percent to 80 percent of the care that physicians can.[1] The doctor provides services—perhaps 10 percent to 30 percent depending on specialty—that only physicians have the training or legal ability to do. Studies over the past twenty-five years have found that NPs and PAs perform as well as, if not better than, doctors for the remaining physician services.[2]

Although both PAs and NPs substitute for doctors in many circumstances, they are two distinct professions. PAs can do anything a physician delegates to them, except as restricted by hospital privileges and state laws. Most PAs are in primary care and to a great extent are trained on the job. PAs are intended to work under the supervision of doctors and to be a doctor substitute.

NPs perform two roles—that of nurse and that of substitute doctor. The traditional nursing role focuses most on caring for the patient (as distinct from treating the disease), and includes complementary services that doctors do not usually do, such as counseling, medical education, self-care training, prevention, diet, exercise, and so forth. In addition, like PAs, NPs serve as substitute doctors.

It must be emphasized that these clinicians are not physicians. Although doctors are legally enabled to train PAs to do almost any task, PAs should not perform services beyond their level of training. The major distinction in most hospitals between doctors and PAs or NPs is that the latter cannot write many prescriptions. However, certain states allow them to perform limited prescription writing, usually for nonnarcotic, noncomplicated drugs.

TRAINING AND PRACTICE OF NPs AND PAs

The occupation of physician assistant was born in the mid-1960s. The first PA program was at Duke University,[3] where I taught a class in the newly established public policy school with Dr. Harvey Estes. He later came to be known as the "father" of the PA movement. The program started with ex-army corpsmen who returned from the Vietnam War with three to six months of medical training. Because there was a perceived doctor shortage at the time, particularly in rural areas, these medics were retrained to perform some of the services normally provided by doctors. The federal government, with an interest in making primary care services available in underserved areas, codified the occupation of physician assistantship, stimulated demand for PAs, and financed their training.[4] Prospective physician assistants without army training undergo about two years of training in medical schools, sometimes taking the same courses with physicians. The emphasis is on primary care.[5]

Nurse practitioners have different training requirements. They are nursing school graduates who go on to receive six months to a year of additional training.[6] Whereas law requires that PAs work only under the supervision of a doctor, NPs are entitled to practice nursing independently from doctors. Each state has a Nurse Practice Act that delineates the requirements and regulations on the scope of practice. Registered nurses in every state are legally authorized to provide care for primary health promotion, disease prevention, and assessment of health status, but different states provide for varying degrees of NP independence, prescriptive authority, and reimbursement.[7] Some states allow NPs fairly wide latitude to perform services without the supervision of a doctor. Independent responsibilities may include diagnosing and managing typical acute illnesses and stable chronic illness, ordering tests, counseling, and sometimes prescribing drugs and treatments.[8] Whereas nurse practitioners can legally accept a fee, physician assistants cannot because they work for a doctor and must be remunerated through the practice.

Unlike the training of PAs, which is directly overseen by physicians, the preparation of NPs is rooted in nursing education, which traditionally is conducted in a separate framework with its own governance and its own sense of itself as a distinct professional calling. This sets up a natural tension between nurses' desire for more autonomy and physicians' desire to control the care offered to their patients. The tension is more apparent when doctors sense a threat that nurses might directly compete with them for patients and for lucrative tasks. This is not unlike the constantly evolving competition between various specialties. My conversations with the experts, presented in Part II, brought me a new understanding of some of these conditions on the ground.

It must be noted that nurses of all educational levels make up the huge bulk of the health care workforce. There are some two to three million nurses working in the United States today. In much the same way that NPs and PAs take on tasks formerly performed only by physicians, nurses are receiving more advanced tasks as well. Consequently, like NPs and PAs, professional nurses are becoming too expensive for some settings. Although part of the problem is direct cost, part of the problem is that nursing schools cannot produce the number of nurses ideally needed because there are not enough nursing faculty. They can be paid far better elsewhere in the system. This means that an enormous number of health workers who could theoretically reduce the need for more physicians are far less available then would be preferred.

GROWING NUMBERS OF NPs AND PAs

Both professions have seen tremendous growth in training program enrollment. In 1990 there were only 4,000 part- and full-time enrollees in NP programs. But by 1999, that number had quintupled to 20,000.[9] Similarly for physician assistants, in 1992 there were only 1,400 PAs graduating, but by 1997, the number had doubled to 2,800.[10]

The increase in training is reflected in the growth of practicing NPs and PAs (see Table 5.1). There were very few NPs throughout the 1960s and 1970s. By 1990 there were 29,000 active NPs, and that number nearly doubled by 1995. The supply of PAs also increased; there were only 11,000 in 1980, quadrupling to 45,000 by 2000. This growth has far outpaced that of physicians. Some projections suggest there will be 170,000 NPs and 100,000 PAs by 2015.[11]

Another startling trend is the relationship between the number of NPs and PAs and the number of doctors. In 1990 there were 18.4 doctors for every NP; this declined to a little over 8 doctors by the year 2000. Correspondingly, there were 28 doctors for every PA in 1990, which declined to 15.8 in 2000. Looking at the forecasts for the number of doctors in the year 2015, we can expect this trend to continue, as I discuss in the next chapter. In that year, there might be 5.4 doctors for every NP and 9.3 doctors for every PA. These dramatic ratio changes underscore the importance of the supply of NPs and PAs within the overall health care workforce.

PRODUCTIVITY AND QUALITY OF CARE

Generally, NPs and PAs provide services that are relatively straightforward, and they call physicians in to examine, diagnose, and prescribe drugs for complex cases. The more routine tasks comprise some 70 percent of services, depending on specialty. It is inefficient for doctors to do those tasks when others can at a lower cost.

Table 5.1. Past and future trends in the number of NPs and PAs, 1980–2015

	1980	1990	1995	2000	2005	2010	2015
Nurse Practitioners		29,000	58,000	88,186	115,000	142,500	170,000
Physician Assistants	11,000	19,000	32,156	45,311	62,000	81,000	100,000
NPs and PAs		48,000	90,156	133,497	177,000	223,500	270,000
Physicians	413,692	532,638	617,362	717,898	802,599	887,300	926,000
Number of Physicians per NP		18.4	10.6	8.1	7.0	6.2	5.4
Number of Physicians per PA	37.6	28.0	19.2	15.8	12.9	11.0	9.3
Number of Physicians per NP and PA		11.1	6.8	5.4	4.5	4.0	3.4

SOURCES: Figures for nurse practitioners for 1992, 1996, and 2000 are from "National Sample Survey of Registered Nurses," U.S. Dept. of Health and Human Services, 1992, 1996, and 2000.

Figures for physician assistants for 1996, 1998, and 2000 are from AAPA Physician Assistant Census Reports 1996, 1998, 2000.

Figures for physicians from 1980 through 2000 are for total nonfederal active MDs from the 2003 Area Resources File.

Figures for nurse practitioners and physician assistants are from R. Cooper, "Health Care Workforce for the Twenty-First Century: The Impact of Nonphysician Clinicians," *Annual Review of Medicine* 52 (2001); R. Cooper, "Current and Projected Workforce of Nonphysician Clinicians," *Journal of the American Medical Association* 280, no. 9 (1998).

Figures for physicians for 2005 and 2015 are imputed from projections given for 2000, 2010, and 2020 in R. Cooper, "Economic and Demographic Trends Signal an Impending Physician Shortage," *Health Affairs* 21, no. 1 (2002).

In some small-group practices, doctors train NPs and PAs to do much of what doctors do. It is important to note, however, that the services and procedures reserved for physicians require additional training.[12] So it is a careful distinction—NPs and PAs are not the same as doctors, although they may perform some of the same tasks.

NPs have begun practicing outside of hospitals and physician offices—often in places that are convenient for people to drop by. At some CVS pharmacies, for example, NPs provide treatment for common illnesses or a referral to a physician for a $60 out-of-pocket fee or insurance copayment. Speed and convenience make such services popular with customers.[13]

PAs and NPs offer about two-thirds of the productivity of physicians.[14] For example, if a solo doctor sees four patients per hour for forty hours a week, the weekly output for this doctor is 160 visits. If a PA or NP is added to the practice, its number of patient visits, on average, will increase by two-thirds to about 266 visits. Typically, the doctor leads the initial visit with a patient,

Table 5.2. Trends in the salaries of NPs and PAs, average net incomes ($2004)

	1994	1995	1996	1997	1998	1999	2000	2001	2002	2003	2004
Physician Assistants			$74,035	$75,219	$74,481	$77,288	$75,425	$75,780	$75,855	$78,064	$78,257
Nurse Practitioners	$63,205	$63,433	$70,288	$67,361	$70,270	$70,349	$67,451	$68,897	$69,433	$73,034	
All Physicians	$216,508	$210,366	$214,961	$219,556	$213,094	$206,632	$206,186	$205,740			
PA Salary as a percentage of Physicians'				34.4%	34.3%	35.0%	37.4%	36.6%	36.8%		
NP Salary as a percentage of Physicians'	29.2%	30.2%	32.7%	30.7%	33.0%	34.0%	32.7%	33.5%			

NOTES: Physician assistant data are for total annual income from primary employer for respondents who work at least thirty-two hours per week at a primary clinical job.

SOURCES: Figures for physician assistants are from AAPA Physician Assistant Census Reports, 1996–2004.

Figures for nurse practitioners are from NP Central, www.nurse.net/cgi-bin/start.cgi/salary/index.html, last accessed April 14, 2004.

Figures for physicians are average net income across all specialties from AMA SMS datafiles for 1993, 1995, 1997, 1999, and 2001.

with some help from the PA, and the doctor makes the diagnosis. Follow-up visits may be entirely delegated to the PA, with the doctor periodically seeing chronically ill patients personally.

There is considerable evidence that the quality of care provided by PAs and NPs is as good as, and in some cases better than, the quality of care provided by physicians.[15] There is also evidence that NPs and PAs have very good patient acceptance.[16] They are used throughout the health care system by integrated HMOs, such as Kaiser Permanente,[17] as I discuss in detail later in this chapter. Not surprisingly, the growth of managed care has increased the demand for PAs and NPs over the past few decades.[18]

NPs and PAs are more likely to practice in underserved areas, probably because they require less population density than physicians.[19] NPs—who in half of the states do not have to be supervised by physicians[20]—have had a big impact on underserved areas, enlarging the health care workforce there.[21] Although PAs must be supervised by a physician, they do not have to practice at the same site. In rural areas, doctors can supervise PAs with a beeper and a phone. Some hospital systems utilize telemonitors so that PAs in outlying locations can communicate with physicians at the main hospitals, especially in emergency medical situations, so that patients can have access to board-certified emergency physician supervision in remote rural areas.[22]

TRENDS IN PAYMENT TO NPs AND PAs

Unlike physician incomes, which fell overall after the introduction of managed care, NP and PA incomes have grown. The differences between their earnings and those of physicians have narrowed. As of 2004, NPs and PAs earn about $70,000 annually, whereas doctors make over $200,000. Table 5.2 illustrates that, although NPs and PAs provide two-thirds of the productivity of doctors, they earn about 36 percent of doctors' average salaries.

Various states have different methods of paying nurse practitioners and physician assistants; each has its own licensing board, Medicaid requirements, payment arrangements, and laws governing NP and PA practice. NPs can bill independently, if the insurance company will cover the fee. Generally, Medicare will pay NPs for services that are within their practice guidelines.[23]

MANAGED CARE AND NPs AND PAs:
CLOSE-UP ON CALIFORNIA

It makes sense for managed care organizations to hire NPs and PAs when they are more cost-effective than doctors. An HMO can pay about three NPs or PAs for the price of one doctor; working together, they would be 33 percent more productive than a single doctor hired at the same price as the three NPs or PAs in total.[24] Of course, it should be noted that not all patients will accept an NP or PA, and will insist on seeing only a physician.

At the macro level, there has been an increase in the growth rate of NPs and PAs, while there has been a decrease in the growth rate of physicians. At the micro level, managed care organizations have recently been hiring more NPs and PAs. We can look at this substitution more closely by examining the Kaiser Permanente system in Northern and Southern California, comparing its physician and NP and PA workforces to those of the state of California and the country as a whole.

Between 2001 and 2004, the United States and California increased their supply of physicians slightly (2 percent and 3 percent, respectively), whereas Kaiser's supply rose 18 percent. At the same time, Kaiser hired proportionately more specialists than either the United States or California.[25] In terms of NPs and PAs, a different picture emerges for this period. The United States had a 20 percent increase, and California had a 13 percent increase, whereas Kaiser increased its supply of NPs and PAs by only 8 percent (see Figure 5.1).

Why? Because Kaiser, as an efficient health care system, responds to economic incentives. As NP and PA salaries approach those of physicians, they become less desirable in economic terms. This creates an incentive to hire doctors—particularly those whose incomes have not risen as much. Moreover, Kaiser now uses more of its NPs and PAs in specialty care because specialists are more expensive; increasing the productivity of specialists makes more economic sense. Kaiser understands these market dynamics.[26]

It is important to recognize that the services performed by NPs and PAs would have to be delivered by doctors if they were not available. Subsequently, any physician supply analysis needs to include them as an integral part of the health care workforce. In 2000, there were 717,898 doctors and about 125,000 NPs and PAs. Using the two-thirds productivity estimate, the NPs and PAs

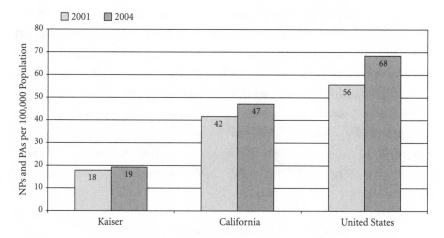

Figure 5.1. Nurse practitioners and physician assistants per capita, Kaiser Permanente, State of California, and the United States

sources: Personal communication with Glen Hentges; and RAND Corporation, "California Statistics: A Service of the RAND Corporation," 2005, available at http://ca.rand.org/ (last accessed on November 10, 2005).

would be as productive as 83,000 doctors. The doctors, NPs, and PAs working together in 2000 produced the same output as 800,000 doctors. This is a very rough calculation; specialty mix is not accounted for, nor is variation among health care delivery systems or the time spent by the doctor in supervision. Nonetheless, even given these caveats and perhaps others, NPs and PAs represent a major, growing, and notably cost-efficient segment of the medical workforce.

OTHER NONPHYSICIAN HEALTH CARE WORKERS

In addition to NPs and PAs, the economy seems to have taken on more nonphysician health care workers. This includes secretaries, nurses, technicians, and many more health professionals. In a more indirect way, these people can help relieve the burden of the physician so that he or she can focus on the tasks that require more specialized knowledge.

Table 5.3 shows the increase in both physicians and nonphysician health workers from 1990 to 2006. The nonphysician workforce has increased by 54 percent during this time period, whereas the number of physicians only increased by 47 percent. By 2006, there were 14.3 nonphysician workers for every physician. This is a large support staff. Hence there seems to be an upward trend in the number of workers per doctor. This indicates that support staff has been absorbing some of the demand for doctors by taking on responsibilities that the doctors once did by themselves.

This substitution may be part of the reason physician wages did not grow as quickly as those in other professions, as discussed in the previous chapter. This productivity increase means that more work can be done with the same number of doctors. More work at the same price leads to lower costs. These changes in the structure of the overall health workforce, and the specific tasks

Table 5.3. Growth in number of physicians and nonphysicians

	Active Physicians	Nonphysician Health Workers	Workers per Physician
1990	559,988	7,650,712	13.7
1991	576,225	8,041,475	14.0
1992	592,934	8,361,866	14.1
1993	610,126	8,643,474	14.2
1994	627,818	8,901,882	14.2
1995	646,022	9,162,878	14.2
1996	663,362	9,429,238	14.2
1997	681,168	9,676,832	14.2
1998	699,451	9,841,449	14.1
1999	718,226	9,972,674	13.9
2000	737,504	10,120,296	13.7
2001	752,842	10,435,258	13.9
2002	768,498	10,767,502	14.0
2003	786,658	11,030,442	14.0
2004	792,154	11,263,146	14.2
2005	807,997	11,505,903	14.2
2006	824,157	11,786,843	14.3

NOTE: For doctors, years with data unavailable were extrapolated.
SOURCES: Health worker data from BLS data series CEU65620000101, subtracting the number of doctors.
Doctor numbers from Department of Health and Human Services, "Health, United States, 2006, with Chartbook on Trends in the Health of Americans," publication No. 2006-1232, Table 106 (p. 357).

designated to doctors, may be an important driver of efficiency.

It must be noted that health care workforce costs are of major concern. Edward O'Neil notes that 60 percent of the cost of care is attributable to the health care workforce.[27] This is especially important in the face of expected rising demand for health workers. The Board of Labor Statistics projects that the nation will need 3.5 million more health personnel in the next decade—in addition to replacing the 2 million who leave their positions. Unfortunately, there is not an adequate number of training slots to accommodate the need, in part because of a growing shortage of specialized faculty.[28]

This problem is acute in California. A new study from the Health Workforce Solutions in San Francisco, founded by O'Neil, suggests that the demand for health workers in the state will grow by 26 percent (versus overall job growth of 16 percent) by 2014. In addition to registered nurses, there will be a large demand for surgical techs, respiratory therapists, diagnostic medical sonographers, and a variety of other workers.[29]

CONCLUSIONS

One of my pet topics in health care is the role of NPs and PAs, and I've written about it for years. They are relatively new on the scene—just a few decades—but they are a particularly visible part of an evolution that probably goes back to the beginning of modern medicine: doctors offloading tasks to free themselves for the more demanding responsibilities that only they can provide (and not incidentally that are more remunerative). Along the way, there's some tension at the margins over scope of practice, autonomy, and money. State laws, union demands, and the dictates of the medical community are always reworking the particulars. But even these rather formidable forces are inevitably trumped by the press of realities in the marketplace—patients, diseases, costs, and revenues.

My overall point is that you can't weigh the doctor supply without taking account of these folks: what they can do and will learn to do in the future; where they are working and for whom; what they are paid and how that's evolving in relation to what doctors are paid; and how many will be trained.

DOCTOR SUPPLY FORECASTS:

MORE OR LESS

As I was writing this book, I was also planning an end-of-the-year barbecue for my staff. We invited everyone, said they could bring a significant other, and asked for an RSVP. Of course, the RSVP count is only an indicator. Some people forget to RSVP. Things come up at the last minute. Spouses back out. It gets even more complicated when you try to figure out how much food you'll need. How many people will have eaten dinner before they arrive at 8 P.M.? How much does the average person eat?

It may be impossible to predict, but you have to come up with a number somehow if you're the one buying the food. I put some bounds on my thinking by deciding on a worst-case scenario and a best-case scenario. I also thought about the attendance at past barbecues. Because the parties have gone well each year, this event gained a good reputation. More people show up each year. Would the trend continue, or had we reached the maximum barbecue-partying retention rate?

One runs into the same kind of troubles when trying to predict how many doctors will be needed in years to come. As with hosting a party, it's best to plan for several different scenarios in order to cover the bases. Even though perfect foresight is impossible, policy requires that stakeholders come up with a number of medical school and residency slots each year.

MOVING TOWARD THE "RIGHT" SUPPLY OF DOCTORS

Today, there are nearly nine hundred thousand actively practicing physicians in the United States. Some experts say that this represents a significant surplus,[1] some say it's a shortage,[2] and still others believe there is a rough equilibrium between supply and demand with shortages in some specialties.[3] Everyone agrees that the goal is to train and field an adequate medical workforce, but how do we know what the "right" supply is for tomorrow's health care system?

This chapter lays out three approaches to calculating the demand for and supply of physicians. The first is a needs-based model based on rate of expected medical need and use. The second is based on economic factors. The third extends the previous models and encompasses the use of physician assistants and nurse practitioners as an integrated part of the physician workforce; this is called the integrated workforce model. This integrated model is a best-case scenario model, because it tells what will happen if the country does a really good job improving the productivity of doctors. Combining this integrated workforce model with the needs-based and economic approaches produces a more useful forecasting strategy than any one approach can achieve independently.

THE NEEDS-BASED DEMOGRAPHIC MODEL

The needs-based school maintains that the physician supply should be geared toward a benchmark number or ratio. This could be the per capita number of doctors in a specific area or in a particular health system. A version of this was done by the Graduate Medical Education National Advisory Committee (GMENAC) in 1980. For their report, experts measured the rates of disease across the population, calculated how many hours of doctors' time it would take to treat those conditions, divided that by the number of doctor hours worked per year, and figured out how many doctors would be needed to accommodate that.[4] Using this method, GMENAC concluded that by 1990 there would be seventy thousand excess doctors in the United States, and that by 2000 there would be a surplus of one hundred forty thousand.

One advantage of the needs-based model is that it takes into account the aging of the population. Older people see the doctor much more often than younger people. As the baby boomers hit retirement, there will be a much greater need for doctors just because of the changing demographic of the population. The GMENAC experts looked at disease rates for different age

Table 6.1. Projections of physician shortages and surpluses using different methodologies

Projections		Short Run					Long Run				
		2006	2007	2008	2009	2010	2011	2012	2013	2014	2015
Supply	Doctors	775,097	788,179	801,859	816,151	831,069	846,306	862,179	878,713	895,923	913,825
Economic Model of Demand	Doctors	668,068	683,422	699,068	715,013	731,261	747,548	764,141	781,047	798,270	815,816
	% surplus	16%	15%	15%	14%	14%	13%	13%	13%	12%	12%
Needs-Based Model of Demand	Doctors	804,150	814,505	824,859	835,213	845,568	853,577	861,587	869,597	877,607	885,616
	% surplus	–4%	–3%	–3%	–2%	–2%	–1%	0%	1%	2%	3%

groups and calculated the greater incidence of such diseases as those age groups grew.

However, the problem with any needs-based or demographic measurement of physician supply is that it disregards the influence of the marketplace by omitting such economic factors as the income of doctors, the price of medical care, and changes in insurance coverage. This type of "yardstick" measurement also ignores changes that will occur in the future: changes in disease patterns, the number of visits needed to treat diseases, cultural attitudes toward treatment, discovery of new treatments and cures, and the emergence of new diseases. Just as important, yardsticks ignore differences across regions, including differences in health care systems, quality, and health insurance availability. Estimates based on yardsticks cannot accurately predict how many doctors the American public will actually need five years from now, even if they factor in the number of new doctors required to offset doctors' retirement, death, and drop-out rates. This calculation is called a loss-and-replacement scenario.

Table 6.1 shows the demand for physicians calculated using both the needs-based model and the economic model. This table also provides figures for projected supply of physicians, which takes into account the current physician base, expected medical residents "graduating," and physician retirement rates. The needs-based model results show that physician supply will be roughly in balance in the years to come. The demand-based model suggests a surplus of 16 percent in 2006, declining to 12 percent in 2015.

THE ECONOMIC MODEL

The fundamental idea of the economic model is that managed care has made the market more efficient and thereby made it possible to calculate physician undersupply and oversupply in a way that was not possible before. It can be used to calculate the number of doctors in the United States (and worldwide) using growth in the economy as the key determining factor.

It is well known that the best single predictor in the growth of health care spending is the rate of growth in the economy.[5] This is especially true for developed countries such as the United States and those in the Organization for Economic Cooperation and Development (OECD).[6] Research shows that for every 1 percent increase in the GNP per capita in developed countries, there is a corresponding increase of 1 percent or more in health care spending.[7] Data suggests that the growing share of GDP devoted to health care is no anomaly, but simply a reflection of the fact that as people get richer, they want to spend a greater share of their income on health.[8] Because of findings such as these, the economic forecasting model relates growth in income (GNP) per capita to growth in the demand for doctors.

Given this, to the extent that people are expected to get richer, policymakers need to account for the extra doctors they'll want in the economy. That's how demand works in an open market economic setting. How much richer people are expected to get is measured using a forecast of GNP growth. Then these figures are used to predict the growth in the demand for doctors.

Table 6.1 gives the projected demand for physicians based on expected economic growth and the doctors needed to keep up with that growth. The baseline projections show a 16 percent surplus of doctors in 2006. This surplus, however, will shrink in the short run as the disease base grows. Indeed, it will

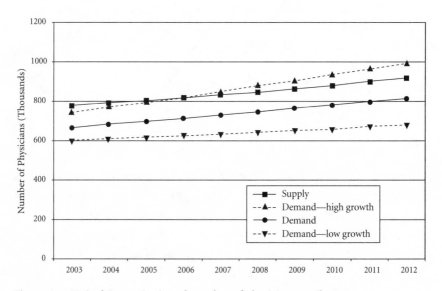

Figure 6.1. United States: Projected number of physicians until 2015

DATASOURCE: Health, Nutrition, and Population database (World Bank), OECD Health Data 2005, World Health Statistics 2006, COGME (2005).

shrink by a full 4 percent by 2015. Keep in mind, though, that these numbers are very sensitive to the difficult-to-predict demand projections. To be conservative, I wanted to include a range of possible demands. Figure 6.1 shows three scenarios that I believe could be likely: high demand, low demand, and medium demand. Because a physician shortage could be more costly than a surplus—at least in terms of price of care—it may be reasonable to err on the high side of demand. In the high-demand path projected in Figure 6.1, there is a slight shortage of doctors, whereas there is a slight surplus in the medium-demand case.

THE INTEGRATED WORKFORCE MODEL

The integrated workforce analysis of the physician marketplace incorporates the concept of an integrated team as the supplier of physician services, not just doctors alone. Economists have suggested the increase in physician support staff as a way of avoiding physician shortage.[9] This would be much cheaper than training more doctors. In particular, I consider the use of physician assistants and nurse practitioners, discussed in Chapter 5.

This model will show how many doctors will be needed if doctors are more efficient than they are today. Chapter 2 explains how managed care forces greater efficiency by reducing fragmentation in the market. The efficiency improvements of managed care have been evident so far. Managed care organizations have adopted creative mechanisms to force doctors to offer care that is most cost-effective.

Of course, it is difficult to tell how much more efficiency can be squeezed out of our doctors. A "best-case scenario" might look something like Kaiser Permanente, one of the best-known managed care organizations. Kaiser provides fewer services, fewer procedures, and fewer patient visits per enrollee than do health plans that provide a great deal more health interventions—yet achieves similar or better health outcomes. And Kaiser does this with fewer doctors and other health workers.[10]

The two main features of my integrated workforce model are that (1) it uses "doctor equivalents" rather than just doctors as a measure of physician supply, and (2) it assumes that the market will drive efficiency all across the country to the same high level as Kaiser Permanente. In other words, it assumes that the nation will only need as many doctors per capita as Kaiser has doctors per enrollee. But let me explain this in detail.

To calculate doctor equivalents, assume that each NP or PA is equivalent to two-thirds of a physician, on the basis of productivity found in prior research. So three PAs would be equivalent to two doctors. In this case, doctor supply will be determined by the total number of doctors, PAs, and NPs.

What is the target number of physician equivalents? Kaiser uses 40 percent fewer doctor equivalents per capita than does the United States as a whole. As an organization on the cutting edge of efficiency improvements, Kaiser can be viewed as a standard or goal for efficient physician ratios. In a perfect world, the nation's health care system would move closer and closer to Kaiser's level of physician equivalents per population. So we would no longer need as many doctors.

Kaiser sets the bar for the rest of the country in part because there are indicators that they have achieved optimal staffing ratios. In 2001, Kaiser had thirteen NPs or PAs for every one hundred doctors. By 2004, the ratio had declined slightly to twelve NPs or PAs per one hundred, which suggests that Kaiser was hiring more physicians than these other clinicians between those years. The opposite was true for the nation in general. Across the United States, NPs and PAs were being hired more rapidly than doctors. This may mean that Kaiser is happy with its NP and PA to doctor ratio. Because Kaiser operates in a very competitive market environment in California, it is likely that this ratio is the "right" or economically efficient one.

This model would forecast a greater surplus of doctors than either the economic or the needs-based model.

There are a few caveats to this approach. For one, the population served by Kaiser may not be representative of the United States as a whole. Kaiser enrollees come from families with at least one working member and have higher average income than the general population. Because income and health are positively correlated, Kaiser enrollees are probably healthier on average. However, this approach aspires to give a lower bound on the number of doctors needed, so a downward bias in this number will not be as problematic.

THE GLOBAL SETTING

It is impossible to fully address the future demand for doctors in the United States without considering international health systems. To gain some insight into the future global demand, I applied the economic-growth-based model discussed earlier to the rest of the world, predicting that the global demand for physicians will be about 12.7 million in 2015 (see Appendix B).[11] Paired with the projection of physician supply, this number suggests that global supply and demand will be roughly in balance by that time.

The needs-based model, however, projects that the world will need only about 3.8 million doctors in 2015. Keep in mind that this is a bare-bones estimate. It is based on a need criterion used by the World Health Organization that asserts that a reasonable global goal is for 80 percent of live births to be attended by a health care worker.[12]

Of course, these worldwide figures overlook the distributional effects. Even if overall supply and demand are in balance, some countries may have more than their share of doctors, while others want for medical care. Table 6.2 shows how many countries would experience a shortage, according to the needs-based and economic-based models. Africa stands out as the area with the most countries likely to suffer a shortage.

Table 6.2. Number of countries in various parts of the world facing pending physician shortages

WHO Region	Needs-Based Model	Demand-Based Model
Africa	32	15
Americas	1	3
Eastern Mediterranean	3	2
Europe	0	10
South-East Asia	3	0
Western Pacific	6	7
World	45	37

NOTE: Shortage is defined as having a projected supply of physicians that meets less than 80 percent of the forecasted demand or need, calculated at estimated means.

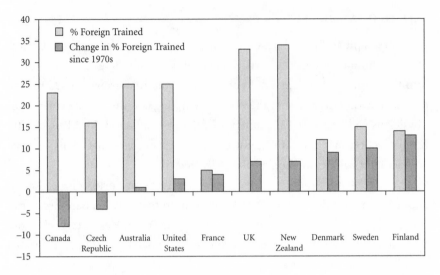

Figure 6.2. Percent of physicians foreign trained

Part of the imbalance among countries derives from the fact that doctors migrate across borders. As a result, countries that pay physicians well constantly have an inflow of doctors trained elsewhere. Figure 6.2 shows the percentage of doctors in each country who come from abroad. Richer countries draw a higher share of doctors in this way. To compound the problem, the share of foreign-trained doctors in high-income countries has increased in recent decades. For example, in a sample of ten high-income countries, eight had seen increases in international doctors since the 1970s.[13] As a result, it can be expected that the maldistribution of doctors will grow over time, particularly given the physician salary differences across countries.

The United Kingdom offers a good example of the cross-country salary effect. Recently England has implemented a pay-for-performance system that allows for higher physician salaries across the board. For example, a primary care physician in the United Kingdom can earn $240,000 under the new system.[14] Compare this with the $163,924 salary for primary care physicians I reported in Chapter 3. Because of the higher price differential across borders, 80 percent of recent growth in U.K. doctors comes from foreign recruitment.[15] As a result, there has been a doubling of foreign-trained physicians in recent years and a tripling of doctors from sub-Saharan Africa.[16] This example speaks for the power of higher salaries to attract doctors across international borders.

Physicians in the United States make more than five times the average salary, as Figure 6.3 shows. At the same time, doctor salaries in other countries have converged to roughly two times the average salary. This naturally draws doctors to the United States, and there doesn't appear to be any trend toward worldwide convergence in this arena.

In general, rich countries draw doctors from poorer countries. India exports doctors at a very high rate. India, Cuba, and the Philippines purposefully train more doctors than they need in hopes that the doctors they send abroad will send money back to their families left behind.[17] Doctors from India make up the largest share of foreign-trained doctors in many higher-income countries. However, many African nations also lose doctors on a net per year basis, simply because the doctors have better opportunities abroad. This exacerbates doctor shortages in Africa, because doctors are leaving as the need for them has been growing.

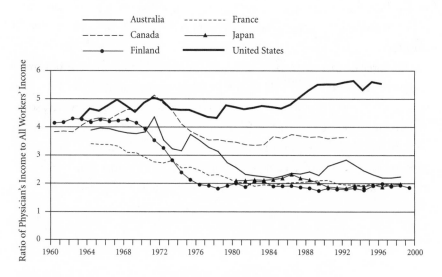

Figure 6.3. Ratio of physician's income to all workers' income

CONCLUSIONS

There are a number of lessons to be learned here. The needs-based model is useful as a guide to evaluate the effect of an aging population on the demand for extra doctors. But in the United States, the market drives things, and as people get richer they also want more doctors, regardless of their health status. The economic model accounts for this effect. By looking at both models, we get a fuller picture of what's going on. Both methods suggest a rough balance of doctor supply and demand. The economic model implies there could be a slight shortage in the high-demand case and a slight surplus in the middle-demand case. Because the population is aging and getting richer, we can assume that more doctors will be wanted over time. If we combined the two models, we might notice a greater demand for doctors than with each model separately, as the effects of aging and becoming richer would be compounded. It is possible, then, to get a slight shortage going forward, assuming that doctors do not improve their efficiency.

However, we have seen that doctors do get more efficient. The integrated model, which includes NPs and PAs, shows that the surplus in the United States in 2006 was 280,000. This is, of course, a calculation based on the Kaiser workforce model, which is of interest, but not realistic for the nation as a whole. However, the potential does exist for movement toward an integrated workforce.

Our forecast for the global market for doctors is crude at best, but quite suggestive. In contrast to the United States, it has supply and demand roughly in balance by the year 2015. Because of unequal distribution, however, some regions face pending shortages. African countries are most likely to go wanting because they do not have the resources to compete with more developed countries to bring in doctors. This point makes it clear that additional resources must be found if Africa is to retain and attract the doctors it clearly needs.

THE "RIGHT" NUMBER OF DOCTORS IN A BETTER HEALTH CARE SYSTEM

Like many Americans, I grew up watching Star Trek. *As a Trekkie, I marveled at how Dr. McCoy, better known as "Bones," was always right when he treated the crew members. He was cranky, irrational, and disliked technology, but he was never wrong. And he had great compassion. He was a true primary care doctor. He was always in the house, or in this case, the ship.*

Fast-forward to a later version of the show, Star Trek: Voyager. *The doctor is now a hologram, or, more precisely, a "volumetric display" that appears at the press of a button. Although nameless, it attempts to show compassion and engage in human interaction, but the advanced technology presents obstacles. This physician has only one thing in common with Dr. McCoy: it is always right.*

This is far-fetched, maybe. But there is no doubt about the advance of medical technology. Technology that saves lives or improves the quality of life will likely be in great demand, as will the doctors who control and deliver it.[1] At the same time, technology that enhances care efficiency—such as electronic medical records—will tend to reduce the number of doctors needed. Both types of technological advances will have an impact on the physician supply cycle, but it is unclear what the net impact will be.

The foregoing chapters lead us to the next step in the Doctor Supply Cycle. It is the most important because it is the only element that we can hope to influence: *Where are we headed?*

But contemplation of the future is unhelpful without applying the lessons learned from the previous stages of the cycle—each of which combines insights from historical and economic analysis. As we have seen, managed care developed and grew in part because of an oversupply of doctors. Doctors were eliciting too high "rents,"[2] so market pressures built until the point when consumers and payers finally demanded a change. Managed care provided that shift and reduced the growth rate of medical care, at least temporarily.

Notably, managed care changed the health care landscape by shifting power out of the doctor's hands. The restructuring of the market changed incentives in a way that allowed for some important improvements. Movements in the income of doctors, geographically and by specialty, have realigned according to the demands of patients and purchasers. Before managed care these things were driven more by doctor preferences. The managed-care-dominated marketplace also affected the racial and ethnic distribution of doctors, and increased the use of nurse practitioners and physician assistants. These clinicians have become a major factor in the size and character of the doctor workforce.

Let us now look at the future. What is the "right" supply of doctors, and what will determine whether that has been achieved? A wide range of opinions can be grouped into two main viewpoints.

IS MORE BETTER?

The first main viewpoint holds that there can never be too many doctors. The proponents of this line of thinking point out that training more doctors is a good idea, especially with an aging population, a growing affluent segment of society, and the need to bring more minorities into the field without necessarily diminishing the opportunities of Caucasian males to become doctors. This was part of the thinking during the dramatic build-up of the physician supply from 1965 to the 1980s.[3]

In economic terms, physicians have externalities. They help both individuals and societies improve their health. The more there are, the likelier it will be that people can have access to one when they have the need. At the same time, a higher quantity of doctors suggests that doctors will have more time to spend with individual patients. (No matter how efficient a hologram might be, people appreciate the painstaking attentions of an actual human being when they need medical care.)

Those who advocate for more production of physicians say it will improve the competitiveness of the system. As in the beginning phases of the managed care revolution, doctors in many parts of the country had no choice but to respond to the cost-efficiency needs of the marketplace. With widespread measurement of physician performance and growing public access to these data, doctors are more likely to compete on both quality and cost-effectiveness measures. To some extent, the more doctors in competition, the better. Another reason for promoting a large increase in the doctor supply has to do with distribution problems, which I have discussed in detail in Chapter 4. Eventually, the thinking goes, physicians will get pushed into rural and underserved areas where their help is critically needed.

The second major line of thinking opposes an increase in the training of doctors for a number of reasons. First, having more doctors does not necessarily lead to better care. In fact, higher competition can lead, and has led, to physician-generated demand. "Overdoctoring," some argue, is more dangerous than "underdoctoring."[4] Other industry observers contend that competition is dysfunctional in health care, driving up costs rather than restraining them, and failing to reward innovation and high quality with consistency. A zero-sum game,[5] the reasoning goes, encourages players to shift costs to the other players.[6]

Another argument, documented in this book, is that the cost of training new physicians is extremely high—around $1 million each (see Appendix A for details). This money might be better spent on improving the performance of the health system. Increasing enrollment would be very costly. The University of Pennsylvania's Richard Cooper, for instance, recommends increasing medical school enrollment by 40 percent by 2015 rather than by the 30 percent that policymakers currently plan on.[7] My calculations suggest such an increase would add 6,370 new medical students each year, which translates into nearly $1.5 billion extra per year just for the undergraduate medical education. The residency training for these additional people would bring the price tag to almost $1.9 billion per year. Because the projections for physician demand are extremely sensitive to uncertainties, this money may turn out to be wasted if we mispredict the tide.[8]

There is also the argument that more services can be had without extra doctors by making the current supply more efficient. For instance, the need for physicians will drop with widespread use of care guidelines, evidence-based chronic care protocols, Internet access to scientific studies, decision-support tools, and electronically based distance care—all of which are quickly improving in quality and ease of use.[9] Another important factor in productivity is the use of nurse practitioners and physician assistants, as I discussed in Chapter 5. The growth in numbers of NPs, PAs, and other clinicians may obviate the need for larger numbers of physicians. The best outcomes will depend on team-based care.

ECONOMIC CRITERIA

In puzzling out conclusions from the differing arguments, it is useful to look to the economic criteria. As we have seen, there has been a dramatic increase in doctors per one hundred thousand people. But that is not a useful criterion. In the denominator, what is really needed is the demand for services for those one hundred thousand people, rather than just the number of people. The doctors-per-capita statistic ignores demand changes. And economic paradigms involve both supply and demand.

Keep in mind also that any economic analysis can take into account the fact that NPs and PAs may substitute for doctors. Chapter 5 explains these concepts in detail. Basically, if productivity can be improved through the use of NPs and PAs, then fewer doctors will be needed, no matter which economic model is applied.

Indicator #1: Rising Incomes

Rapidly rising incomes can be one indicator of a physician shortage, showing that demand is increasing more rapidly or slowly than the supply of doctors. Assuming that there was an appropriate balance of doctors in the recent past, then rising incomes show there is a shortage and falling incomes suggest a surplus.

I believe that the United States had a good balance of doctors somewhere around the year 2000. In the early 1990s policymakers projected doctor surpluses. In 2006, the Association of American Medical Colleges projected shortages.[10] Because we didn't hear much about surpluses or shortages during the time in between, I tend to believe that this time period had the "right" amount from a policy point of view. Also physician wages neither rose nor declined very much around this time. This indicates to me that demand was not putting pressure on the workforce in either direction—for more doctors or for fewer. That's what I call equilibrium.

This viewpoint is bolstered by historical trends. Table 7.1 gives some data on the recent growth rate of physician incomes compared with the growth in incomes across all professions. It becomes apparent that the physician incomes either have grown more slowly than other professions or else have actually fallen over this time period.

On the surface, suppressed wage growth would indicate that the country may be in surplus. However, it's important to put these figures in context. As discussed in Chapter 5, the economy has taken on more nonphysician health care workers. These workers have been absorbing some of the demand for doctors by taking on responsibilities that the doctors once held themselves. It seems likely that physician salary growth has slowed as a result.

This indicates that the nation's need for doctors going forward may depend greatly on the ability to substitute nonphysician personnel for doctors. If the

Table 7.1. Recent growth in physician incomes

	Incomes				Growth Rate (percentage)
	2002–2003	*2003–2004*	*2004–2005*	*2005–2006*	
All workers*	$30,420	$30,980	$31,790	$32,800	2.5
Professional and business service workers*	$34,060	$34,510	$35,570	$37,000	2.8
Radiology	$344,876	$356,724	$365,811	$351,000	0.6
Anesthesiology	$315,502	$318,504	$312,227	$306,000	−1.0
Surgery	$263,281	$263,296	$262,765	$272,000	1.1
OB/GYN	$257,841	$256,926	$254,522	$234,000	−3.2
Psychiatry	$176,246	$174,115	$181,360	$174,000	−0.4
GP/FP	$158,839	$155,005	$154,568	$145,000	−3.0

NOTES: *Using December-January averages wage figures from BLS data series CES0500000000 and CES6000000008. Annual salaries were determined assuming forty hours per week, fifty weeks per year of work.

SOURCE: Physician figures are obtained from Merritt, Hawkins & Associates, "Summary Report: 2006 Review of Physician Recruitment Incentives."

optimal ratios of doctors to support staff have been reached, there could be a shortage going forward. If productivity can be improved in this way, then there is probably the right number of doctors.

Indicator #2: Return on Investment

One can also look at the return on investment (ROI) to suggest whether there is a surplus or shortage of doctors. The ROI is a measure of how much output is received in future physician services from every dollar invested in medical education.[11] The ROI of medical education can then be compared to the ROI of other types of education that high-skilled workers may choose instead of medical school, which leads to the question, Is it worthwhile to train another doctor, or would it be better to put that person through law school instead?

This method looks at the broader context, not solely the market conditions of the health care industry. It makes comparisons across several markets, so it controls well for macro-level factors in the economy, laying groundwork for asking big questions such as, Is this the best way to utilize the nation's resources?

I conducted an analysis of ROI to physician training. Table 7.2 shows the results of the analysis, and how these figures vary over time (see Appendix A for details). As physician incomes have risen, so has the return on investment. It rose almost two full percentage points between 1982 and 2001, for instance. I must place the ROI numbers in context, however. Lawyers earn a 25.4 percent ROI, dentists earn a 20.7 percent ROI, and a graduate business degree will bring a return of about 29 percent.[12] Note that the ROI for doctors is less than for lawyers and businessmen, but more than for dentists.

What can we learn from comparing the ROI across professions? The first thing to notice is that doctors have a lower ROI than other professionals. A

Table 7.2. Return on investment for physicians, as percentages

	All Physicians	Specialists	GPs
2001	20.2	22.7	18.8
1993	21.1	24.3	18.5
1983	18.3	20.5	17.4

large part of the difference comes from the fact that medical training costs a lot more and lasts longer for doctors than for lawyers or business professionals. In fact, given the difference in training costs, it's remarkable that doctors still enjoy a 20 percent ROI. It is worth noting that even though the ROI for medicine is lower than some other highly professional degrees, it is still a very good investment. The rate of return on general education (such as high school and college) is only about 8.5 percent per year.[13]

Comparing across professions also helps put the medical ROI into perspective over time. In 1978, I wrote a paper on the medical ROI with Roger Feldman.[14] At that time we found a 22.0 percent ROI in 1970. I find it remarkable that this figure has not changed very much over time. When you look at the difference in ROI across professions, you realize there's much more variation than in the ROI over time. This implies that investment in medical education is a *safe* investment. Imagine you were trying to invest in a stock. If you found a stock with a 20 percent rate of return and very little long-run risk, you'd probably jump at the opportunity to buy that stock.

What does the ROI story say about the supply of doctors? The medical ROI is high compared with general education and compared with other types of investments, such as stocks. The ROI is also very stable. It doesn't vary much over time. These things imply that it's worthwhile to train the doctors that are currently being trained. As a nation we could probably even train a few more and still enjoy the high return on investment. I'm not saying a sound ROI is cause to cry "shortage." But it certainly means that training more doctors won't be difficult. These returns would surely produce applicants for medical schools.

QUALITY DISTRIBUTION AND EQUITY ISSUES IN SUPPLY

If there is a difference in the quality of care across doctors, there could be equity issues in access to care. After all, a top surgeon has only a certain number of hours in the day to perform surgery. Not everybody can be treated by the country's "best" surgeon. Of course "best" may be difficult to define, but reputation and measurable outcome success can be important factors.

What determines the lucky patients who get treated by the number one doctor? One train of thought says that top surgeons can make more money by accepting only the highest-paying patients, those with private, fee-for-service insurance. However, many surgeons may value things besides money. For instance, renowned surgeons often work at medical schools. These doctors may value the academic environment and the social responsibility of treating lower-income patients. In either case, many people who need the surgery must be treated by a doctor who isn't the number one surgeon.

When does quality distribution matter? If high-quality doctors are financially selective (accepting only high-paying insurance), then low-income people will consistently face lower-quality medical care. This could lead to health disparities. Similar disparities could arise geographically if people located close to a medical teaching hospital have better access to care. Income and geographic disparities can both have an impact on quality of care.

This quality distribution issue can actually suggest whether or not more doctors are needed. Here the question is, Are the least-in-demand doctors sufficient for treating the lowest-access people? Doctors in high demand may have long wait times. But as my informal survey of San Francisco restaurants showed, this fact is uninformative in assessing physician supply. If the lowest-access populations (say the rural poor) have long wait times, then there is hint of a physician shortage.

HOW TO PROCEED

Paralleling many of the preceding arguments are two principal schools of thought about what needs to be done. The first is a case for a modest increase in the training of doctors. The second school argues that the current supply is adequate, but must be better distributed by location and specialty, and also needs to be deployed in more efficient ways to produce better quality and consistency.

The other idea of improving the system within a market is to give patients incentives to choose high-quality, low-cost providers. This requires giving physicians incentives that are aligned accordingly. For example, doctors could be tiered so that patients who choose high-performing doctors would have lower or no copayment or deductible. In other words, as Michael Porter and Elizabeth Olmsted Teisberg put it:

> The way to transform health care is to realign competition with value for patients. . . . If all system participants have to compete on value, value will improve dramatically.[15]

To make this happen, they argue that performance measurement and the reporting of results is central to the improvement of the health care system.

There's a fundamental problem with this approach. At its essence, health care is local and personal. We will never get away from wanting a Dr. McCoy who is not only right but who convinces us that he cares. As pointed out by David Mechanic:

> Despite its size and sophistication, American medicine is built around local markets and culture, and a highly individualized perspective. The public thinks in terms of personal stories and anecdotes and not in terms of populations and statistics. We go to great lengths to save individual lives at enormous cost and with great compassion, but we care much less about policy initiatives that save many more anonymous lives at much lower cost.[16]

His major concern is that a health care system needs to be built on trust—people have trust in their medical group or hospital, and they also have trust in their individual doctor. The economic considerations in weighing the physician supply do not include the element of trust. So there is a conflict between the production model, which is about efficiency, and Mechanic's emphasis on trust.

Nevertheless, virtually all health system stakeholders and expert observers agree that the system is broken and needs to be fixed. Americans are not getting enough good health outcomes from the health care dollars we spend. And yet, we could. In his compelling essay "My Right Knee," health quality leader Don Berwick sets out the five things that he and all patients require from our care providers: no needless deaths, no needless pain, no helplessness, no unwanted waiting, and no waste.[17] It seems obvious, yet nowhere in the United States can all of these be found today. Nevertheless, Berwick assures us that each of these necessary conditions exists right now in particular organizations across the country. He names names. The strong implication is that excellent care on all five dimensions is within reach.

To what extent is fixing health care a social responsibility? Alice Rivlin and Joseph Antos remind us that health care spending is projected to rise above 20 percent of all American spending by 2015, according to the President's Council of Economic Advisors. They talk about the market versus the regulatory approach:

> Proponents of regulation argue that just because regulation has sometimes been carried out stupidly does not mean it cannot be done well. They envision a system

of universal health coverage in which the government uses its power to ensure that health services are effective and delivered efficiently. This could involve analyzing data to establish best practices, promulgating practice guidelines, and refusing to pay for care that did not conform to those guidelines, as well as imposing caps on total health spending and devising roles for enforcing those caps.[18]

Nevertheless, Rivlin and Antos recommend a blended approach to reform—neither wholly market-based nor wholly regulatory.[19]

Finally, I agree with Stephen Shortell's call for the reframing of health care policy efforts as "a search for value and new ways of creating value." According to Shortell:

> [V]alue creation is shifting from investment in tangible assets of physical capital to the intangible assets of human capital, information, and knowledge capital and customer relationships. . . . [T]he current primary emphasis on cost containment as a way of creating greater value will give way to a greater emphasis on quality and outcomes of care as we realize the huge value leakage resulting from unneeded costly variations in clinical practice and error rates and defects in treatment that would not be tolerated by most other sectors of the economy.[20]

For its part, the Institute of Medicine, with its far-reaching Quality Initiative, has recommended a broad redesign of the health care system that includes a framework to better align incentives relative to payment and accountability for quality.[21]

ONE ECONOMIST'S VIEW

How does this economist view the future? As the health care system expands and the population ages, there is good reason to expect that the nation will require more physicians. The baby boomers are going to need more doctors when they develop chronic conditions. The groups that use the most medical care will be growing very rapidly[22]—more rapidly than the number of doctors. At the same time, the needs-based model discussed in Chapter 6 accounted for the age-demographic changes, and this model still projected a rough balance by 2015. However, if this model is off base, even by a little bit, the problems could become magnified as the population ages.

The degree to which the present doctor supply will be able to keep up with this increase in demand will depend greatly on how much more productivity can be gotten out of the physician workforce. Basically, it's a race between the increasing demands of a growing elderly population and the increasing efficiency gains from better technology and workforce structure. If these two forces do not offset one another, physician supply will fall out of balance.

As an optimist, I feel there is still some hope that we can further integrate the workforce. Teams of doctors, nurses, NPs, and PAs can work together to meet some of the pressures of the oncoming demand. This integrated workforce model—which would resemble the Kaiser Permanente system—could be especially useful in primary care and in underserved areas.

Moving toward an integrated Kaiser model has many challenges, however. Legal and regulatory changes are indeed slow, and they may be needed in some parts of the country. The habits and culture of medicine are even more formidable as potential barriers to change. Economic factors are always in play. Health care delivery is quite local, and a one-size-fits-all approach is sure to fail.[23]

As the country moves into the future, we will have to watch for the potential ways to expand capacity. To err on the safe side and make us less dependent on international medical graduates, I do recommend a 10 to 20 percent increase in the number of U.S. medical students over the next decade. I think it's also important to focus on the other avenues for expanding capacity. Physician assistants and nurse practitioners are taking on responsibilities not only in primary care, but also in some specialties as well. Other nonphysician providers will also need to be deployed. I expect this to continue as increasingly sophisticated decision-support tools take more guesswork out of the diagnosis and treatment areas. One can easily imagine an expanding role for nurse practitioners and physician assistants.[24] New medical technology is clearly the wild card. Gene-mapping, stem cell research, new drugs, and other developments all have promise for increased health. Given the determination of Americans to pursue good health, it can safely be assumed that they will be willing to spend more and more to achieve and maintain it. David Cutler, in his book *Your Money or Your Life*, makes a convincing case that one should spend more on medical treatments because Americans value life and are willing to pay for it.[25] We will see.

I believe it is better to err on the side of too many doctors than too few. Too many doctors means money has been wasted on training unneeded people. Too few doctors means people will go untreated for medical necessities. It also means that underserved populations, such as the poor, will suffer to a greater extent. That's not acceptable. This recommendation, however, must go hand-in-hand with a call to improve efficiency. Improve the nonphysician support for physicians, improve the use of IT, improve the geographic distribution of doctors, and encourage primary care practice with financial and other incentives. These things must accompany any decision to increase capacity.

Strategy for Implementing Policy

How should we as a society go about creating the modest increase I have suggested? To expand capacity, we must consider both graduate and undergraduate medical education. Expanding internship and residency programs is usually the first place to look. For one, residents and interns provide services, so they can directly alleviate some of the demand for medical services. We can also expand graduate medical capacity fairly easily in the short run by bringing in international medical graduates (IMGs) to fill those spots. Currently there are 224,042 IMGs (2004 data) and 884,974 total physicians.[26] The actual number of U.S. citizens graduating from foreign medical schools is unknown, but 4,186 U.S. citizens registered for Step 1 of the U.S. Medical Licensing Exam in 2002.[27]

Subsidizing residency spots can help to expand capacity. Such incentives are a powerful tool governments use to guide young people into careers that will pay off for society in the long run. An example from my own experience was the launch of Sputnik by the Soviet Union. when I was about to enter college. Concerned about a perceived shortage of future scientists, the National Science Foundation started seeking out good math students like me and offering scholarships for taking science courses. The extent to which the United States should employ subsidies for medical residents is the subject of ongoing debate.

The Balanced Budget Act of 1997 capped the number of resident physicians that Medicare would subsidize. To some degree, residency spots have continued to increase, despite the cap. This happened because the residents provided valuable labor to the hospitals. But if we want the number of residents (and hence the supply of doctors) to increase faster than the current rate, we will have to subsidize the market.

Resident subsidies also offer a solution to some of the distribution problems discussed in Chapter 4. Relative to the demand for services, there is some misdistribution across specialties. Also, too few medical students choose to go into primary care practice when they graduate. This shouldn't surprise us. We know that specialists make more money in the long run. In other words, primary care and a few particular specialties may be suffering because of the financial incentives currently in place. The government can offset these problems by subsidizing the less popular fields. These educational subsidies can be a cost-effective way of addressing long-run problems.

So in the short run, we can expand residency positions and bring in international medical graduates to fill whatever spots Americans don't take. In the long run, however, it's probably best to grow our own doctors from scratch. By importing doctors from abroad, we may exacerbate shortages in developing countries.

Expanding undergraduate medical slots in the United States is more complicated than expanding residency spots. Should we expand the number of slots in existing medical schools? Or build new medical schools? Building fresh medical schools involves high fixed costs. As a result, the average cost of adding more students through new medical schools is high. We only need to consider marginal costs when adding more students to each medical school.

Of course, the pecuniary costs do not account for other factors. For instance, larger medical school classes may mean a lower quality of education for each student. Medical school requires a lot of hands-on training, which could be stretched thin if too many students are present. Such factors have to be weighted against the cost when it comes to expanding capacity. In practice, this probably means assessing each medical school separately to see how many extra students can be added without decreasing quality.

Industry Standards and Efficiency

Industry standards provide a necessary protection from market forces. Without standards, quality could wane in response to the demand for cost cuts. However, industry standards can also be used by insiders as a way of maintaining rents[28] and high profits. Because government standards lie outside the grasp of the market, it is government's responsibility to make sure that standards appropriately balance quality with efficiency.

I've discussed the $1 million it takes to train a doctor. Much of the cost comes from the high standards required for physician training. Medical industry insiders have a strong hand in determining medical school standards. From an economic standpoint, this is somewhat problematic. Doctors have the incentive to keep too many people from becoming doctors. When competition is low, doctors can enjoy the higher salaries that go along with a limited supply.

The obvious way of limiting the number of doctors would be to limit the number of spots in medical school. Indeed, that happens. A more indirect approach is to keep the cost of training very high. This way, even if the government wants to add more doctors, it is difficult and costly to do so. To counterbalance industry interests, policymakers have to be constantly on the lookout for industry "standards" that are inefficient or wasteful.

As it is, undergraduate medical students learn to conduct their own medical research. How important is it for a doctor to know how to conduct research? I have a joint appointment in the Goldman School of Public Policy here at the University of California, Berkeley. We teach our public policy students to read and interpret serious economic research. But we do not teach them to conduct their own research. They can think critically about what they read, but they cannot necessarily produce their own new economic model. Economics doctoral students spend an extra three years in training and learn to do the hardcore modeling. We don't feel that's necessary for the policy students. We give them only what they need in order to make informed decisions. This situation could be analogous to that of doctors. If doctors want to keep up with the latest medical research, they need to know how to read and interpret the studies that come out. Unless we want doctors conducting research in their practices, we may be investing too much money in teaching them research skills.

Training standards are not the only avenue for doctors to regulate the field. There are vast differences in the "allowed" responsibilities of NPs and PAs across states.[29] I have shown the potential efficiency gains from greater utilization of nonphysician personnel. Managed care has driven greater substitution in this area. But regulations on prescriptive authority and other practices can counterbalance the push toward efficiency. In areas where NPs and PAs have shown proficiency, regulators need to make sure that legal standards do not inhibit them.

The point here is that policymakers have a responsibility to look for areas where industry interests may be trying to protect rents. Monitoring standards is one avenue through which doctors protect rents. This is an avenue untouchable by market innovations such as managed care. As a corollary, it deserves special attention. These matters will have direct impacts on the number of doctors we need, so they must be considered in tandem with the standard problems of supply and demand going forward.

A "Flexner Report" for the Twenty-First Century

In the end, it will be up to policymakers to make choices on behalf of Americans in terms of the physician supply. It will not be easy. Victor Fuchs notes the various explanations for the collapse of the Clinton health plan in 1994—that it was poorly explained, had a flawed political strategy, and succumbed to special interests. He says these things probably played a role, but that the fundamental reason for the failure of the plan was "the unwillingness of policymakers and the public to make the difficult choices that are inevitable if the U.S. is to improve its approach to health care."[30]

As they engage in the decision-making process in the areas of doctor supply and training, our policymakers should give thoughtful regard to the 1910 report by Abraham Flexner.[31] This carefully devised document assessed how medical education needed to be changed and restructured. It recommended a heavier focus on the scientific method, and standards of training and licensing doctors in accordance with scientific proficiency. The report carried tremendous influence in the direction of medicine for decades following its publication. Preparing a "Flexner report" for the twenty-first century could prove an opportunity to shape the doctor supply in ways that would benefit all Americans.

This new report might include new rules and education not only for physicians, nurse practitioners, and physician assistants, but for the entire health care workforce. To focus only on a segment of the workforce may be a good first step toward ensuring an adequate or appropriate supply. But a comprehensive consideration of all health occupations is ultimately the better approach.[32]

Much can be learned from national experiments such as the health care team models used in the military. The physician assistant occupation grew out of lessons learned in the military. Numerous approaches that have been tried in other countries are worth a careful look. To take one example, nurses in the

United Kingdom have recently expanded their scope of practice and can now provide many services that had previously required doctors.[33] This is a topic for another book.

CONCLUSIONS

The lessons that have been learned since the passage of the Medicare Program in 1965 indicate clearly that the supply-demand balance does change and sometimes quite rapidly. My sense is that the physician workforce is about to be hit in some key places where pressure has built. Some physician specialties will no longer exist five to ten years from now. Their function might not be needed or almost completely precluded by technology and other health workers.

New technology will require science-based team models. Physicians will work more closely with Ph.D. holders from the sciences and biotech firms to discover and deliver care.[34] The aging of the population and the explosion of chronic illness will present another shock to the health workplace. There will be dramatic increases in the demand for physicians, nurses, and other health workers to care for the elderly. Work on this needs to begin now.

Though the evidence I provided shows that the spatial distribution is being improved by the market, there will be continued need for workforce models that can be applied in rural isolated areas. I feel very positive about the expanding use of telemedicine. Continuing to diversify the workforce along ethnic and racial lines is a good thing for patients and society as a whole.[35] Understanding the language and culture of patients will improve the quality of care delivered.

Broadly available and affordable health insurance is of course crucial to the health of Americans. But it is only part of the equation. True improvement will require integrated reforms throughout the system. To do this will require behavior and culture change within the field of medicine, as well as on the part of health systems, payers, and patients.

II

CONVERSATIONS WITH THE EXPERTS

Part I of this book puts forward a data-driven view of factors related to the doctor supply. As an economist, I understand the value of these things, and I believe the quantitative analysis helps to illuminate the issues. But I wanted to present readers with a richer understanding of the issues by discussing them in depth with experts representing a wide variety of perspectives.

The following twenty-seven conversations are not intended to serve as qualitative research. Rather, they are reflections of the wisdom of leading professionals in health economics, academic medicine, health systems, advocacy organizations, policy bodies, and foundations. Many are practicing physicians in addition to their teaching, research, management, and policy work. Several have an M.B.A. or M.P.H. as well. Most are on the front lines of health care training and delivery, and the energy of those environments comes through in their words. As can quickly be seen from these fascinating, freewheeling exchanges, these individuals were not selected because they agree with me. In fact, some lively debates on the issues are included in full.

Most gratifyingly, these experts were willing to go beyond their research and to explore with me their hopes and expectations for health care delivery and the physician supply going forward. Therefore, many of the ideas that are included have not been published anywhere. Indeed, despite having been in health care academia for many years, I learned much from these experts, and that is what I wanted to share with readers. Then, in "A Final Word," I attempt to synthesize the lessons from my own research and analysis with the combined wisdom represented in these conversations.

To begin, I called on my colleagues in health economics, then sought perspectives from the front lines of medicine, academic training, and policy.

TOWARD TIERED HIGH-PERFORMANCE NETWORKS

ALAIN C. ENTHOVEN, PH.D., is the Marriner S. Eccles Professor of Public and Private Management, emeritus, at Stanford University, and a core faculty member at the Center for Health Policy and the Center for Primary Care and Outcomes Research. He was a founder of the Jackson Hole Group, a national think tank on health care policy.

RS: You have been called the "father of managed competition" for your work in rethinking the health care system within the competitive framework. What's wrong with the fee-for-service system that supported individual physician practices for so long?

ENTHOVEN: Essentially, modern medicine is a team sport. We can't tolerate a lack of coordination anymore because it's too expensive, technology is expanding health care, and the population is aging and living with chronic disease rather than dying.

> Essentially, modern medicine is a team sport. We can't tolerate a lack of coordination anymore.

Just to give you an example of uncoordinated fee for service, I met a man recently who had atrial fibrillation. So his cardiologist did the normal thing and put him on a blood thinner. The problem is, the doctor had no way of knowing that the man had a history of bleeding ulcers. He was hospitalized and almost didn't survive.

RS: So an integrated system like Kaiser could handle this better?

ENTHOVEN: It wouldn't have to look exactly like Kaiser in California. For example, in Colorado Springs, Kaiser is working with solo doctors. And the Marshfield Clinic in the middle of Wisconsin does that. They have an extended network. The Mayo Clinic's primary care clinics are linked electronically to the mother church. So they can take X-rays and send them back to the radiologist in the central office.

RS: I visited Mayo a few years ago and was particularly interested in their rural delivery with nurse practitioners. The nurse practitioners are linked in with the doctors electronically, and they manage patients that way.

ENTHOVEN: I think that's the future. However, I would not go so far as to say that the whole problem could be solved there. It may be that we need more doctors. But it's got to be efficient. What I'm calling for is for everybody in

America, from sea to shining sea, to be in a model where everyone has a range of responsible choices—some group-practice-based HMOs, some IPAs, some PPOs, and some fee for service. And let those who choose the most efficient alternatives keep the savings.

RS: **What will it take to get us from where we are now to that kind of world?**
ENTHOVEN: Let me start with the beautiful state of Wisconsin, whose legislature recently passed a proposal called Healthy Wisconsin. It would give everybody the kinds of choices that state employees have—which is twenty-three plans to pick from, and the state pays for the low-price plan. About 90 percent of state employees are in HMOs. A payroll tax on employers and employees would capture the amount of money that they are paying to their insurance companies. That amount would be brought into a central pool, which would allocate a premium credit to every resident of Wisconsin—enough for the low-price plan.

RS: **How would the delivery systems and the solo doctors react?**
ENTHOVEN: It helps that Wisconsin has several highly reputable, physician-led delivery systems. Also, there are some other systems that could start offering their own prepaid plans. So I think that medical groups would start offering their own medical plans, which amounts to per capita prepayment because they commit to get the job done for the premium revenue. A lot of doctors who are now in fee-for-service solo practice would see where their patients were going and would take another look at joining a group practice. They'd have a good IT system, and they wouldn't have to fight all the practice management problems.

RS: **What would be the role of the private health insurance industry? Is this an attempt to put them out of business in Wisconsin?**
ENTHOVEN: No. I see several roles for them. One is to team up with multi-specialty group practices to offer private-label health plans. For example, in the more competitive days, there was a Lahey Clinic / Blue Cross HMO in Massachusetts. Healthy Wisconsin would accelerate a movement toward tiered high-performance networks and capitated primary care networks. In fact, I think a promising model would blend the two.

RS: So patients would have incentives like lower copays to pick more cost-effective providers?

ENTHOVEN: Yes, the doctors would be sorted by quality and by cost per case. That steers people toward the cost-effective doctor. However, cost per case and cost per capita are very poorly correlated, and a system like that could ignore primary care, disease management, and disease prevention. A good model would have tiered high-performance networks, and also capitated primary care networks. You'd steer the business to the specialists who produced cases at lower cost, and pay them by case.

> A good model would have tiered high-performance networks, and also capitated primary care networks.

RS: What are the drawbacks to this combined model?

ENTHOVEN: The specialists would be working for several different companies, so building a good IT system would have to involve a lot of doctor input and be doctor-friendly. Also, there would need to be a point-of-service plan.

RS: How would this new market model work?

ENTHOVEN: Michael Porter's idea of competition is based on what he calls integrated practice units.[1] Out there someplace in Berkeley, you've probably got a back pain clinic and a diabetes clinic and a coronary artery disease clinic. But these are separate entities. They don't talk to each other and share records. So the integrated comprehensive care systems are a lot better because all of the doctors taking care of you are partners and use the same guidelines.

RS: The business schools don't push that.

ENTHOVEN: Yes, business schools tend to like multispecialty group practice. Porter doesn't like that bundling because he says people should be able to go to the best orthopedic team, unconstrained by their network. Of course, if we applied that to business schools, students could get their finance courses at Wharton, their accounting at Stanford, and so forth.

RS: It would take a long time to get a degree that way.

ENTHOVEN: Right. Laura Tollen and I wrote an article replying to Porter.[2] I think there are important advantages to integrating the system. The insurance companies would compete with physician-sponsored delivery systems with their own health plans, like Marshfield Clinic, or maybe like the California delegated model. There are challenges, though, with two hundred medical groups up and down the state, and they all contract with seven insurance companies. With pay for performance, if one of the carriers greatly improves the performance of the medical groups, the benefits are shared across all seven health plans.

RS: So it's the free rider issue.

ENTHOVEN: Right. We want all the carriers to contribute a substantial amount of money to the reward pool, but some of them do and some don't. You just don't get incentive alignment the way you do in Kaiser, where there's a genuine partnership between health plan and medical group. There it's simple: what the Kaiser doctors want to do is what's covered. The medical group understands that the health plan is not going to survive and prosper unless the rates are competitive, and the health plan understands that they're not going to survive and prosper unless the doctors are really good. So they have to bring in enough revenue to pay really good doctors. There's a mutually beneficial partnership, and I just don't see that happening with the California delegated model.

RS: How should the P4P money be spent?

ENTHOVEN: There are two camps in the Integrated Healthcare Association. There's the "social Darwinian" camp, which says we just pay for the best. And then there's the "social democrat" camp, which says you've got to help the weakest to improve. The reason the health plans want to do it is to see better quality scores, and you have more leverage over scores if you focus where there is the most room for improvement.

There's the "social Darwinian" camp, which says we just pay for the best. And then there's the "social democrat" camp, which says you've got to help the weakest to improve.

RS: When it comes to scores, patients don't use them to select providers do they?

ENTHOVEN: Patients don't use them a lot, but I don't think that necessarily matters because doctors are A students. They want to get good grades.

This was the experience in New York with bypass graft surgery. The results did not move market shares or patient flows, but they caused something to happen among the doctors and the hospital boards. I remember a very heart-warming story about the "worst doctor" in New York and the "worst hospital" in New York. They did a lot of data analysis and figured out exactly how and why they were performing poorly compared to the best hospitals. Then they changed their processes and soon were among the better hospitals. In the process, some low-volume, poor-performing doctors were forced out.

PRIMARY CARE AND THE MEDICAL HOME

KAREN DAVIS, PH.D., an economist, is president of The Commonwealth Fund, a national philanthropy engaged in research on health and social policy issues. She served as a deputy assistant secretary for health policy in the Department of Health and Human Services in the late 1970s. She is a member of the IOM Committee on Redesigning Health Insurance Benefits, Payment and Performance Improvement Programs, and serves on the Panel of Health Advisors for the Congressional Budget Office.

RS: **The Commonwealth Fund, which recently published very interesting reports[3] on the American health care system, also compared it internationally. What did you find out about what Americans are looking for in their health care system?**

DAVIS: People are frustrated with the complexity and fragmentation. Nine of ten people yearn for one medical practice that knows all there is to know about them. They want all their information in one place and accessible to all of their doctors. What they're describing is the medical home model, which lines patients up with a regular doctor and a regular practice that is accessible by phone and has the patient's comprehensive medical information. Patients can get in the same day; there's coverage on nights and weekends. Care is coordinated.

Nine of ten people yearn for one medical practice that knows all there is to know about them.

RS: **Can you differentiate the medical home from the earlier vision of primary care?**

DAVIS: There was always a philosophy of primary care as offering a long-term relationship with patients, easy accessibility, referrals to community resources, and help with coordination of care. But I think managed care created problems by introducing some mistrust. Patients began to worry that doctors might deny them something because they were being paid to deny it. The gatekeeper model is not what people want.

RS: **Did that affect the length of the doctor-patient relationship?**

DAVIS: Yes. Because of the instability in coverage, a lot of people got into the

mind-set of changing doctors regularly. About half
of people change physicians within three years,
mainly because they changed jobs or the employer
changed the plan. When we do our international
studies, we find that Americans are much less likely
to have the same doctor for five years or more.

About half of people change physicians within three years, mainly because they changed jobs or the employer changed the plan.

RS: **So that's another reason why primary care is not an attractive specialty.**
DAVIS: Yes, the financial reward is not as great, and there's a perception that
the hours will be long. It doesn't work if you want work-family balance.
So the shortage of primary care doctors is helping bring about the medical
home concept.

RS: **Do you think that the electronic medical record allows this to happen in ways that it couldn't have happened before?**
DAVIS: Absolutely. You can't fulfill all the functions of a medical home with-
out it. I like to tout the Danish system, in which 98 percent of the PCPs have
a totally electronic system. There's a health information exchange so that all
that information goes to a nonprofit organization called MedComm. When
a doctor orders a prescription, it flows through MedComm, and when the
patient picks it up at the pharmacy, MedComm electronically notifies the
doctor. So you always have an active medication list of filled prescriptions.

RS: **In the standard practice in the U.S., a doctor doesn't know whether a patient fills a prescription. Or even whether a patient has different prescriptions from different doctors.**
DAVIS: Exactly. Plus the Danish system has a comprehensive program for
off-hours care. From 4:00 P.M. to 8:00 A.M., there are doctors on phone banks
taking calls from patients. They can pull up your information and prescribe
medication immediately.

RS: **The U.S. is far behind other countries in terms of the electronic medical record and other types of data management.**
DAVIS: It's shocking. Most of the major European countries are at the 90 per-
cent rate in terms of electronic medical record keeping, whereas the U.S. is

down around 20 or 25 percent. Of course, in some of these countries, the government paid for it.

In Denmark, physicians buy their own software, although the government sets standards and also funds the information exchange. That way, providers never have to worry that they're buying a software system that will be antiquated or won't work. Twenty or so software companies sell products, so you can buy any of them and be able to interact with MedComm.

RS: In addition to managing data better, what should we do to improve health care in this country?

The first key to change is extending health insurance to all.

DAVIS: The first key to change is extending health insurance to all, although some people worry that we can't cover everybody if there aren't enough doctors to provide even the care needed now.

The second idea is organizing the care system to be able to provide accessible and coordinated care. That is partly the medical home concept, but it also means having linkages to specialists. We have to think about incentives that will encourage integrated delivery systems to grow, rather than contract. In addition to Kaiser Permanente, there are other models of care.

RS: Can you give me examples?

DAVIS: The Geisinger Health System in Pennsylvania has 650 salaried physicians, of whom 200 are in primary care—many of them practicing in three- or four-person primary care clinics spread over a forty-county area. Geisinger is now moving to multispecialty clinics as well. In addition, there are convenience clinics at night, staffed by nurse practitioners. Everybody's on the same IT system. Because it's a big system, all patients can be referred on if necessary to somebody else within the system.

We went to North Dakota in July, where there are shortages of pharmacists. So they use pharmacy techs who are backed up by video-conferencing with pharmacists a hundred miles away. The pharmacist actually sees the prescription on the screen and can allow the tech to dispense it through pharmacies all over the state.

RS: **What are your thoughts about the best ways to pay providers?**

DAVIS: In terms of a lever for change, I like the blended or bundled payment that includes medical home monthly fees. Primary care physicians are paid a mix of fee for service, monthly patient panel fees, and bonuses for performance on quality and efficiency. Then for acute inpatient care, it's a bundled fee that includes physician and hospital services, as well as ninety days of post-hospital care. Geisinger charges a single fee for coronary bypass surgery, and it offers a warranty. If you have to go back into the hospital, it's all covered by the same fee.

> *Geisinger charges a single fee for coronary bypass surgery, and it offers a warranty.*

RS: **Do you think the nation should move toward larger, more integrated systems?**

DAVIS: Yes, and seeing these models in rural areas in Pennsylvania and North Dakota, you realize you don't need a huge building. You can have integrated systems that are in smaller facilities, decentralized into communities, but all connected by being part of an organization.

It can be attractive to primary care. Geisinger does not think they will have a problem recruiting primary care physicians, nurses, and others. They can offer a setting where the off-hours are taken care of and salary is guaranteed. They have a lot of joint programs with nursing training in order to get people trained and to stay in the local area.

RS: **How can we make these ideas work within the market model?**

DAVIS: I envision a level playing field. We need to make Medicare work, with its Medicare Advantage plans on an equal footing with what I think of as the Medicare self-insured product. This gives people choices. The plans would be paid comparably, rather than with the differential that exists now. For example, Geisinger offers their own managed care plan, as well as fee-for-service care. So you can join the managed care product and only get your care from Geisinger hospitals and doctors, or you could be in the self-insured product and get some of your care in other places. The competition is not so much among providers as it is competition between a self-insured public program and private managed care plans.

RETHINKING THE FINANCING OF GME

GAIL WILENSKY, PH.D., is a senior fellow at Project HOPE. She is an elected member of the Institute of Medicine and has served two terms on its governing council. From 1990 to 1992, she was administrator of the Health Care Financing Administration, directing the Medicare and Medicaid programs. She chaired the Medicare Payment Advisory Commission (MedPac), and testifies frequently before Congressional committees.

RS: You've spent a lot of time on the GME [Graduate Medical Education] issue, and you've said that we should pay the indirect costs. Those costs were added when prospective payment was put in and it happened to be correlated with things we wanted to pay for like uncompensated care.

WILENSKY: I think we should pay for the indirect costs because it costs more for a hospital to have GME programs on board. Otherwise seniors won't be able to access academic health centers.

I think we should pay for the indirect costs because it costs more for a hospital to have GME programs on board. Otherwise seniors won't be able to access academic health centers.

RS: So by taking a lower-than-market wage, these residents are paying their tuition.

WILENSKY: Exactly. It has been hard to knock out the excess subsidy. And, politically, that's not very attractive. It's similar to the discussion I have with people about why having health care funded through employers and not the government doesn't make firms less competitive. What makes firms less or more competitive is their productivity and the total labor compensation—not the distribution between cash wages and fringe benefits. Of course, the employers say, "No, no, no. What makes me less competitive is that I have to pay health care costs while people in countries with national health insurance don't."

RS: Right, the government pays for it.

WILENSKY: And the fact that they pay higher taxes doesn't seem to enter people's thinking.

I believe the current delivery system is going to be driven to change because the spending is unsustainable. The rewards are going to be toward more consolidation of the institutions and physicians involved in the patient's care, either real or virtual.

RS: **Right. In California we may be looking at just two huge systems over the next ten or fifteen years.**

WILENSKY: What is especially important is getting the physician groups together with the hospitals, because that's the unit that's providing care and it allows for much more accountable health care groups. The way it is now, there are a la carte patient visits for a particular event, when it should really be about the ongoing treatment of a chronic disease. Even the people who do bypass surgery or other high-cost, high-volume interventions—those are the groups that you'd like to hold accountable, not trying to judge quality by each individual encounter.

RS: **Do you support pay for performance?**

WILENSKY: Well, if you use that term in the most loose, global sense it's fine. It's one strategy. I also support value-based insurance—rewarding the comparative clinically effective work. If you start rewarding the institutions and physicians who are producing high-quality care in a lower-cost way, all the structures and systems change.

However, if you're talking about the more narrow concept of pay for performance a la the Integrated Healthcare Association of California, I don't think that will produce the changes the system needs. That approach looks too much at process, and that's not going to begin to drive enough change.

The more narrow concept of pay for performance . . . I don't think that will produce the changes the system needs.

RS: **Do you think there is an impending shortage or surplus of doctors?**

WILENSKY: If doctors continue to practice as they do now and remain primarily in small, single-specialty groups, there is likely to be a shortage. But if the practice style is like those at the Mayo Clinic, it is not at all obvious there will be an overall shortage.

RS: Do you mean we don't have to worry about the supply right now because there's enough slack in the system for the next ten years?

WILENSKY: We have other things we need to worry about first that will affect the desirable supply. We have unsustainable health care spending with serious quality problems. How we fix that will affect the supply. There is some slack in the system, or at least a lot of efficiencies that could be achieved if the pressure were there to make that happen.

WHAT THE MARKET SIGNALS ARE SAYING

MARK V. PAULY, PH.D., is the Bendheim Professor and chair of the Department of Health Care Systems in the Wharton School at the University of Pennsylvania. He is a professor of health care systems, insurance and risk management, and business and public policy at the Wharton School, and a professor of economics in the School of Arts and Sciences at the University of Pennsylvania.

RS: Do you think we have a shortage or surplus of doctors?
PAULY: That depends on how you define a labor shortage. I believe you use a "dynamic shortage" definition in which undersupplies in broadly competitive markets are signaled by rising prices and profits.

RS: I do. What definition would you use?
PAULY: Two other definitions may have some relevance. The first is the no- tion of government-caused price control shortages. This is the standard econ text rent control model. By putting a lid on prices paid to suppliers, the government creates excess demand. In the health care workforce, this has not been true of physicians yet (with the possible exception of Medicaid), but is being predicted by some doctors for Medicare if Congress does not raise fees rather than go along with the scheduled reduction. The private practice phy- sicians I know well say this time they are going to walk away from Medicare patients, and they really mean it.

The other definition of shortage is based on a cartel-inspired contrived scarcity. This is the Friedman-Kuznets story. They calculated the rate of re- turn on education for physicians and dentists, and proposed that the higher return for doctors was the result of the American Medical Association's im- position of restrictions on entry.[4] In other words, doctors were able to protect their own market environment quite successfully.

RS: I do agree that the government can create a shortage by paying below market rate as you suggest. The market that has suffered shortages is Med- icaid, as you note. This is the reason why I suggest that a small surplus of doctors might be justified so this market is not overlooked. It would also keep up the competitive pressure on prices.

I calculated the rate of return to medical training, and it is still quite high—over 20 percent, and it has changed very little over the past twenty-five years or so. This is clearly the result of heavy subsidy given to the training of doctors. The matrix is somewhat complicated because of supplier-induced demand.

PAULY: As you know I am not a believer in demand inducement to any serious extent. First, I think the evidence alleged to support it is usually weak. But also, it lacks logic: If demand inducement at the margin is important, why are physician incomes or their rates of growth finite?

RS: I would say incomes are finite because the doctors are afraid that policy-makers would come in and regulate them if incomes were too high.

PAULY: In any case, I believe the flood of new medical grads in the 1970s and 1980s wiped out any cartel effect, if it ever existed. Physicians may not have been affected so much by changing market equilibria as they were by the movement from monopoly to competition.

RS: My perspective is that changes in physician supply paved the way from monopoly power to competition. The oversupply enabled managed care to get a foothold by offering a countervailing force to the market power of physicians, bringing strength to the purchasing side. My empirical work supports the notion that there was balance around the year 2000. What do you think of that?

PAULY: I think there is a lot of plausibility to that, but it is my perception that the groups within medicine who captured the power to interpret workforce data shifted. In the 1990s it was academic physicians who defined what I would call a normative non-economic surplus. In effect, they said, "We have more doctors than we 'need,' regardless of whether consumers want them." These days Buz Cooper and Tom Getzen have captured the field with a demand-based model, as opposed to a need-model.[5] My main point is that the change between 1990 and 2010 may have been largely a change in self-styled workforce experts' perception or interpretation of the facts, not a change in the facts themselves. I am programmed to think of markets for doctors—or nurses for that matter— as potentially working as ordinary efficient markets. This is desirable. One labor market that is pretty efficient and responsive to market forces is the market for health care M.B.A.s or M.H.A.s, which I know well. The number of applicants of a given level of qualification ebbs and flows with aggregate demand.

RS: When I worked at the University of North Carolina, I found out how quickly training program applicants do respond to incentives. Changing the fellowship stipend by 10 percent caused students on the margin to change their plans and move to or from a school.

PAULY: The problem with doctors and nurses is that they are produced domestically in an academic market that does not seem to behave like a real market. Instead there is a shortage of places relative to the number of qualified applicants, and marginal tuition appears to be below marginal cost. The cartel-conspiracy theory suggests that tuition does not rise to clear this market because prices that are less than cost provide a way to justify a limited number of places. In addition, there is the whole issue about filling in with international medical graduates. The real glitch in medical labor force markets is in the supply of training. I am not optimistic that this can work better.

> *My sense is that the economic or policy forces needed to change things are not present right now. The public likes having doctors.* [RS]

RS: You're right. My sense is that the economic or policy forces needed to change things are not present right now. The public likes having doctors and trusts them to do the right thing.

RESIDENTS, PAYMENT, AND THE GLOBAL MARKET

JOSEPH P. NEWHOUSE, PH.D., is the John D. MacArthur Professor of Health Policy and Management at Harvard University. He heads the Interfaculty Initiative on Health Policy and chairs the Committee on Higher Degrees in Health Policy. He is the founding editor of the *Journal of Health Economics*, serves on the Board of Health Advisors of the Congressional Budget Office, and has been a member and vice chair of the Medicare Payment Advisory Commission (MedPac).

RS: **We know Medicare pays the direct cost of GME as the salary plus money for training. What can you tell me about the way the indirect cost payment works?**

NEWHOUSE: The payment is based on the estimated coefficient of residents per bed in a regression of cost per case on residents per bed and other variables. The current indirect payment uses a figure well above the actual regression coefficient, and that excess is a subsidy. Moreover, the coefficient seems to fall over time roughly in proportion to the increase in residents, indicating the relationship is not causal.[6] In other words, there's something about the product of the teaching hospital that is correlated with the number of residents, but the number of residents itself doesn't causally increase cost.

RS: **What might it be measuring if it's not quality?**

NEWHOUSE: Well, it's mostly not measuring case mix. I had the MedPac staff run an analysis of what would happen to the coefficient if you expanded it to 900 DRGs, as CMS is now proposing to do. That's a more accurate measure of case mix, but the coefficient hardly budged.

RS: **So if it's not the case mix, what is it?**

NEWHOUSE: I think it's just a different style of care. People talk about the standby capacity, but I still think it's mostly just a different product for the same patient. It's the fact that you have a resident there at 2:00 A.M. when the patient has a crisis, and he gets treated differently than if the nurse calls up the doctor at home and says, "What do I do?"

RS: Right. I'm not sure it's any better, but it's certainly different. Would you agree with the assertion that the relative value scale, which is obviously based on service intensity, is not good to primary care doctors in Part B?

NEWHOUSE: I just wrote an editorial about that in the *New England Journal.* It discusses what happened to the distribution of Medicare patients by type of service and specialty in the first ten years of the RBRVS. It shows that the fees for primary care service evaluation and management (E&M codes) went up 20 percent, but the share of physician revenue going to E&M is constant.[7]

RS: Do you think pay for performance will change the system?

NEWHOUSE: My general view of P4P is that we're in the early days and there's probably too much hope invested in it at the moment. How much change also will depend on how much pay is at stake. In terms of the amounts involved, the U.K. is way ahead of us.

RS: In this country, we get a lot of our primary care doctors from among the IMGs [international medical graduates] who come here to train. Some people say this amounts to a "brain drain" on countries that badly need their doctors.

NEWHOUSE: I don't think the right way to address the brain drain is to erect trade barriers. First of all, in Africa, and probably in Asia and India as well, I think that many Western-trained M.D.s will treat the elite anyway. As with oil, it's a world market. So I'm not sure the ethical argument is so potent. Should we feel badly that they're caring for people in the U.S. if the alternative is caring for wealthy people outside the U.S.?

Should we feel badly that the IMGs are caring for people in the U.S. if the alternative is caring for wealthy people outside the U.S.?

PHYSICIAN INCOME AND THE POTENTIAL OF P4P

UWE E. REINHARDT, PH.D., is the James Madison Professor of Political Economy, and a professor of economics and public affairs at the Woodrow Wilson School, Princeton University. He has been a member of the Institute of Medicine of the National Academy of Sciences since 1978, and is a past president of the Association of Health Services Research. He served as a commissioner on the Physician Payment Review Committee, established in 1986 by Congress.

RS: **You've said you don't think we should pay any federal money for GME. Why not?**

REINHARDT: When I spoke to Congress about that, I said, "I'm going to do two things. First, I'm going to convince you that there is no economic case for having GME at all; second, I'll ask you not to yank it until you've covered all the uninsured. If you yanked it now, you would really traumatize the hospitals financially because they rely on this cheap labor. Jim Knickman wrote a paper on what it would cost a New York hospital to replace GME with physician assistants and nurse practitioners.[8] It was full of hugely boring statistics, but basically it said the NPs and PAs (1) only work forty hours a week, and (2) get paid more.

RS: **Right, residents work far longer and for less pay.**

REINHARDT: It's bad enough for a nation to tolerate having so many uninsured. But we then exploit the most vulnerable group in society—residents. They have four years invested in medical school, and then they have almost no choice except to become indentured labor in order to finance health care for the uninsured. Working them to death, ruining their marriages and their health, is the most despicable thing a nation could do. No one has been able to convince me that it's necessary for a young physician to work thirty hours in a stretch in order to get a good feel for a case. Anyway, look at how risky that is for patients. You don't let a pilot fly a plane or a truck driver drive under those conditions. Why would you let somebody who hasn't slept for thirty hours put chemicals in people's bodies?

Why would you let somebody who hasn't slept for thirty hours put chemicals in people's bodies?

The workforce piece I would worry about more is nurses. I don't understand why this country doesn't build more nursing schools. A lot of medical centers don't want to have anything to do with it. The number of young women who want to go—and men now—have a hard time finding a slot.

RS: In the wake of the managed care revolution, do you think the market will go back to more supply-induced demand?
REINHARDT: My view would be no. The managed care of the 1990s was aggressive in its treatment of doctors, reducing them to dependence on contract rates. This was a model that massively ticked off doctors, and it is probably not going to survive, because in the process, you tick off patients. But it will have to come back in some new form because with open-ended fee for service you'll give away the checkbook.

So one looks for a new managed care model to see who manages it better, where the physicians actually get paid rather well and they really manage the care, and now there's this idea of the medical home.

RS: Do you see the medical home as a model that should be pushed?
REINHARDT: I do. It's a way for the primary care doctor to oversee the electronic health record of the patient and, in the process, become that person's care manager instead of being the gatekeeper. It's a quite different role.

RS: What about the pay-for-performance part of it?
REINHARDT: Well, it can't be a piddly amount. Recently, a member of an IOM panel on P4P proposed the idea of paying something like $100 a year per patient to maintain that person's electronic health record. While she was presenting, I noticed her Blackberry lying on the table opposite me, and I posted, "With all due respect, I've never been more underwhelmed." Now if you pay them $500 a patient, that's going to add up quickly and they'll probably do it.

I view P4P as a two-by-four by which you get the attention of hospital boards, and even doctors. If you sit on a board and hear that P4P is coming down, you've got to take this quality stuff seriously. Before P4P, quality was kind of like the flag; you saluted, then completely forgot. If you pay the hospital a differential of

I view P4P as a two-by-four by which you get the attention of hospital boards, and even doctors.

2 percent for quality, it doesn't seem like a lot. But with a margin of 3 to 4 percent, which is what these hospitals have, it could probably impact the cost by 30 to 40 percent just by doing 2 percent on the top line. When it comes to doctors, you'd have to put some real big money on the table. It should be "pay for performance," but it should *also* be "no pay for no performance."

RS: **You've indicated that you don't believe we have a shortage of doctors. What is your reasoning?**

REINHARDT: First of all you have to break the numbers down by specialty and then look at the context. In the tightly managed systems like Kaiser, you can report about eight hundred to nine hundred patients per physician because of the way they deliver care and use auxiliary personnel.

RS: **That's the model Jonathan Weiner used when he predicted 38 percent of physicians would be without work by the year 2000.**

REINHARDT: Right. The other school of thought was that the tightly managed group or standard model HMOs wouldn't ever spread much in America. We would use physicians fairly clumsily, and therefore we'd take care of maybe four hundred to five hundred patients per physician. So it depends on what world you model.

RS: **Then there's the Richard Cooper school. I spoke with him personally about this, and he is a clear proponent of expanding medical school and residency capacity.[9]**

REINHARDT: Right, Cooper looks at the correlation between the demand for physicians and GDP, which is a remarkably tight correlation, as is health spending per capita and the GDP.[10] You could say the number of physician visits per capita over time actually decreased. At one point it was 4.8, but it's lower now. The aging of the population doesn't really drive it that much now. So what do you need all those physicians for?

RS: **Well, Cooper's is a derived-demand hypothesis, obviously. GDP drives spending, and you can't spend without having doctors.**

REINHARDT: But you do have to take into account price effect and also how doctors make their income. A lot of doctors now derive income from tests or capital equipment, and, of course, the hollowing out of the hospitals.

In terms of demand, Jack Wennberg found that patients in the last year of life use vastly different numbers of physician visits. And within that, the numbers of specialty versus GP visits are hugely different.[11] The demand for physicians is so elastic, so flexible, that almost anything goes. In my doctoral thesis, I looked at the physician-population ratio across the U.S., and the number is just enormous.[12] It varies, but it's very large. Then I looked at the visits per physician produced and that varies pretty much to countermand the variation of physicians. Physician visits per capita didn't vary nearly as much. Interestingly, visits were ten to fifteen minutes, and they have increased a little bit. So while doctors were whining that they couldn't provide long visits because of the HMO demands, David Mechanic[13] quietly pointed out that the average length of visits actually increased from fifteen to seventeen minutes in the 1990s.[14]

RS: Do you think that, under managed care, we got a better set of market signals to look at shortages and surpluses of doctors rather than the ratio work that you did?

REINHARDT: Well, it also has to do with physician-induced demand. Places like Boston or Washington, D.C., would have too many doctors, right? They could just jimmy up the number of revisits, and also do a lot more things per visit. Other places had relatively fewer doctors, and they had shorter visits and not as many revisits.

But with all the problems we have with American health care, that's the one I worry about the least, because if we control the demand side halfway reasonably, we'd obviously have too many doctors. They'd just make less income.

MEASURING PERFORMANCE: HOW AND WHY

PETER R. CARROLL, M.D., is chair and Ken and Donna Derr-Chevron Distinguished Professor, Department of Urology, University of California, San Francisco. He is also associate dean of the UCSF School of Medicine and director of strategic planning and clinical services for the UCSF Comprehensive Cancer Center. His work focuses on cancer induction, progression, and care.

RS: What is the impact of P4P on the specialties?

CARROLL: Looking at individual practices, I can see that the specialties are all really unique—almost cultural microcosms of activity. The way people in different specialties actually measure their work using similar metrics is quite variable, amazingly so. A recent article in *JAMA* showed that P4P may have the least tangible impact on behavior—much less impact than we once thought.[15]

> The way people in different specialties actually measure their work using similar metrics is quite variable, amazingly so.

RS: There was quite a spirited response to that paper.

CARROLL: Yes, there was a flurry of letters that were very insightful. A few issues stood out for me. First, I think P4P on paper sounds very good. It makes sense. It has external validity from the population perspective, and that resonates well. But we have to be careful that we don't take low-hanging fruit, focus on things that are easily measured but probably do not translate into major health benefits. At the same time, measurement shouldn't be so burdensome or difficult that we spend more time trying to measure something than we do actually changing behavior.

Another concern is that people might be tempted to manipulate data or put systems in place that simply change a metric without translating into better behavior. This could occur as a result of public disclosure about performance. One could look at case comorbidity or complexity, and start to refer patients one way or another based on the expectation of more adverse outcomes in one patient population over another. This is a selection effect, and it was seen in cardiac surgery.

Last, the incentive has got to be significant and important to the provider, to the patient, and it has to be culturally or socially valued.

RS: **An example of that in your field would be?**
CARROLL: For surgeons, two performance metrics are the use of prophylactic antibiotics within one hour of surgery, and deep vein thrombosis prophylaxis. These are important, and focusing on them has changed behavior, not because of economic benefits to surgeons, but because these data are increasingly public and that moves people to act. One problem with P4P is that any financial incentive may flow back to the department in academic institutions, the health care industry, but often not to individuals providing the care. People have to be at risk for their performance.

RS: **The typical process involves a withhold. Say 5 percent of the gross revenues might be withheld, and then that's distributed among groups or departments in some fashion.**
CARROLL: Yes, and I think that the institutions have to value these things. They can't scoff at them. That value has to be transmitted carefully and consistently across the medical center.

RS: **How will you keep this information top-of-mind for the doctors?**
CARROLL: Well, what I'd like UCSF to do is to have a Web portal where my individual report card pops up in the corner, so I see it on a daily basis, and it's benchmarked against others. I think people will do the right thing. Unfortunately, at times, rewards may be given to people who go from being poor to good, not good to great, and not staying great consistently.

> *I'd like to have a Web portal where my individual report card pops up in the corner, so I see it on a daily basis, and it's benchmarked against others.*

RS: **What are the kinds of things you hope will change?**
CARROLL: Certainly I'm seeing behavior among physicians that may be costly and not helpful. I'm seeing the rise of entrepreneurial methods of compensation. For example, a physician group buys the local surgery center, purchases a radiation machine and a CT scanner, and derives revenue from ancillary services. I believe we didn't see this so transparently before. We'd be better

off, I think, putting more money and time into preventive services, health behavior modification, community health planning, and so on.

RS: **Nurse practitioners are becoming a bigger part of the workforce, and they're getting more expensive. How are they compensated at UCSF?**
CARROLL: Our NPs make very good salaries actually, and they're going up. They perform great services to patients in unique and very productive ways. The hope is the NPs are taking things off the physician's plate. At UCSF we measure all our physicians' relative value units (RVUs). The remarkable thing is that it's very different across specialties.

RS: **I suppose you've found that there are two things going on here. One is the complementarity. The other is the substitute ability.**

> *There are two things going on with the use of NPs. One is the complementarity. The other is the substitute ability. [RS]*

CARROLL: I thought that there would be a strong ratio between the use of NPs and departmental, clinical activity. After controlling for the total number of bodies, this falls down. So it is not the case that the use of NPs routinely results in that physician doing more to the degree that you'd expect. I see wide variation in that.

RS: **Let's talk about GME and the two-part Medicare payment system. How do you figure out which is the training part and which is the service part?**
CARROLL: It's not as metrically driven as I'd like. One thing we wrestle with is that, in organizations, the doctors are compensated for their clinical effort, whether it's in administration, or paperwork, or patient care. Here at UCSF, we have a large component of effort such as education and research, which is clearly part of who we are but is very poorly compensated.

RS: **What would you do about educational debt? These young doctors are faced with trying to pay back their debt at the same time they're starting a family, buying a house, and all of that.**
CARROLL: I am concerned about increasing debt and the effect it may have. I hear from young physicians who are steering away from academic medicine for higher-paying positions because of it. Programs that forgo or reduce such

debt for service should be expanded. On the other hand, I see a lot of BMWs in the parking lot.

RS: **You could say that medicine still has a strong pull as a profession.**
CARROLL: In fact, it amazes me when I hear physicians complain about their lives. It is a wonderful life. We get to meet remarkable people and do remarkable things. I went through residency and I was up many nights. There is paperwork. But we do things that other people don't get to do. We get to know people in a way that you really can't otherwise. The opportunity to change health care is sitting right in front of us, and we need to seize the opportunity.

PAYING FOR PRIMARY CARE IN AN OUTMODED SYSTEM

JORDAN J. COHEN, M.D., is president emeritus of the Association of American Medical Colleges (AAMC) and chairs the Arnold P. Gold Foundation, which advances humanism in medicine through innovations in medical education. He is a former member of the Special Medical Advisory Group of the Department of Veterans Affairs, and has chaired the American Board of Internal Medicine and the Accreditation Council for Graduate Medical Education.

RS: Do we have a shortage of primary care doctors?

COHEN: The availability of primary care services is critical because the disease burden is becoming more heavily skewed toward chronic, persistent, unremitting illness and disability. For patients to have a "medical home," as many people are advocating, requires a set of skills and a consistent relationship across time that I don't think other kinds of specialists can really provide.

RS: I demonstrate in my book that when the market shows a preference for certain specialties—say radiology—these market signals show up in medical school student preferences. Have you found that to be the case?

COHEN: Yes indeed. The interest of medical students in primary care careers over the past couple of decades responded remarkably quickly to the waxing and waning signals from the market over that time. It gives one some hope that if the market could be made more attractive for primary care, then we'd again see an upturn of interest among U.S. graduates. Medicare, obviously, is the eight-hundred-pound gorilla, and its policies are reflected pretty quickly in other payers. But even after the market signals change, it would take a while for the supply to reflect it just because of the length of time it takes to fully train a physician.

What if we suddenly found a cure for cancer and a way to prevent all heart disease? We might not need so many new doctors.

RS: What can you tell me about the balance between U.S. medical graduates and foreign-trained ones?

COHEN: Today, most of us are predicting a major shortage of physicians for the future. But what if we suddenly found a cure for cancer and a way to prevent all heart disease? We might not need so many new doctors. We have a 25 percent buffer factor in terms of foreign medical graduates in GME. So there's plenty of room for us to overshoot the mark simply by substituting U.S. graduates for foreign-trained ones.

RS: Do you think we should continue to rely heavily on IMGs?
COHEN: There are some countries, India perhaps being the prime example, where they are consciously educating physicians for the export market, so at least they claim not to need all the physicians that they're educating. But in sub-Saharan Africa, the emigration of physicians to other countries is a bloody disaster; the same is true for other parts of the world, as well. So I don't see the justification for a rich country like ours depending so heavily on other countries to educate our physicians.

RS: Well I've talked to others who point out that it's a global market and people have the right to go where they want. That's the case for engineers, scientists, poets, Nobel laureates. Why should doctors be different?
COHEN: One important reason is that medicine is a local phenomenon. If you don't have doctors in Ghana, you can't just buy your medical care on the open market.

RS: What do you think about American medical students studying abroad?
COHEN: Many of us were largely indifferent of that problem when we thought we were training more than an adequate number of physicians. But if there is an impending shortage, it's almost a moral obligation to accommodate the aspirations of more well-prepared U.S. citizens, rather than consigning them to medical schools elsewhere that we know are not as educationally robust.

RS: Of course there's been a lot of growth in osteopathic schools, and the great majority of those graduates go to the same residency programs. There are about five thousand grads now.
COHEN: You're right, osteopathic graduates are increasing much more rapidly than are allopathic graduates and are beginning to compete for limited clinical learning venues. It could turn out to be a pretty ugly confrontation. For several years now, many of us have been seeking ways to heal the historic

breach between the two medical professions in the U.S. In the final analysis, for one country to have two medical professions doesn't make a lot of sense.

RS: **What are your thoughts on financing health care?**
COHEN: We need to move toward prospective financing of large, integrated delivery systems that are accountable for the outcomes of care for a large, defined population.

RS: **Are you describing, to some extent, an integrated model like Kaiser?**
COHEN: Yes, and also the VA. Those are two examples of an integrated, coordinated system of care. They can do a tremendous amount in the way of improving quality, cutting costs, reducing workforce demands, and increasing patient safety. But the cultural changes for physicians are going to be huge.

One of the things that I've been preaching for some time is that the system isn't broken. If it were just broken, we could find ways to fix it so it worked like it used to. It's not broken. It's outmoded. It's a legacy system that never was designed to deal with the kind of problems that we have now. We need an entirely new design.

If the system were just broken, we could find ways to fix it so it worked like it used to. It's not broken. It's outmoded.

RS: **Well, it was designed in the nineteenth century.**
COHEN: Right. It did reasonably well when cost escalation wasn't a big deal, when there wasn't much that doctors could do anyway, and when it was mostly acute, self-limited disease that didn't require long-term coordination of care. Also, safety issues were not as big a problem, and the technology wasn't so sophisticated and difficult. So all the factors that allowed fragmented, small units of accountability to function no longer exist. We now need much larger units of accountability to deal with the large, systemwide challenges of today.

ADVANCED-PRACTICE CLINICIANS
CHALLENGE TRADITIONAL MODEL

TRACEY O. FREMD, NP, is a reproductive endocrinology and infertility nurse practitioner. She works with underinsured Californians at Mar Monte Planned Parenthood, Sacramento. She is a member of the Advisory Board of the Access Through Primary Care Initiative of the University of California, San Francisco, and is a past president of the California Association for Nurse Practitioners (CANP).

RS: **Are nurse practitioners moving from primary care to specialty care?**
FREMD: Nurse practitioners have the biggest fiscal impact in specialty practice. For example, nationally, a noninvasive cardiologist median salary is $280,000, depending on experience and location. An experienced cardiology NP's salary is approximately $70,000 to $95,000 per year, and clinically the services provided by the NP overlap 70 to 80 percent of the services of an office-based cardiologist. The ob/gyn physician median salary is $250,000, while an NP salary is $70,000 to $95,000, and there is a 90 percent overlap in clinical practice in the office. This general rule applies to most specialty practices. In primary care practice the salary tension is a bit greater. The national median salary for physicians is around $160,000. Nevertheless, family practice and other primary care settings continue to be the largest models that utilize NPs in the nation.

Nurse practitioners have the biggest fiscal impact in specialty practice.

RS: **How do you figure the overlap?**
FREMD: It can be estimated by a number of methods, although it's somewhat subjective. Two I use are also used within Kaiser Permanente in Northern California. First, when physicians or advanced-practice clinicians are hired, regardless of specialty, a list of "core competencies" is signed off by a proctoring physician. We find that the list is identical for advanced-practice clinicians and for doctors.

Second, we look at the electronic schedule templates that are used for doctors as well as for advanced-practice clinicians. Most are identical in numbers of patients seen, appointment types, and appointment time allotments.

Exceptions are made, particularly in the specialty practices where the physician blocks a long appointment for new patient consults.

RS: My calculations suggest that, on average, the NP or PA services overlap with those of physicians by about 66 percent.

FREMD: I've heard this estimate, and don't think it's accurate because it assumes that NPs and PAs spend a third of their day chasing down an M.D. consult or referring someone to a specialist. We'd quickly be out of a job. When utilized in the proper way I think the overlap is much more than 80 percent or even 90 percent with an experienced NP or PA. I admit that it is an emotionally charged topic because the traditional model of health care delivery is changing rapidly.

Of course, all methods of estimating overlap are somewhat subjective because definitive numbers don't exist. Our model includes in-office M.D. consults for "out of scope" advice and specialist referral. Data on specialist referral can be misleading because, for instance, an NP in gynecology might refer a patient for a skin cancer evaluation; this would not be within the NP's scope of practice but would nevertheless constitute a referral in an electronic database.

My sense is that doctors tend to be sympathetic to expanding the PA role and much more negative about expanding the NP role because they can be viewed as more direct competition. [RS]

RS: My sense is that because of the supervisory role that doctors have with PAs, they tend to be sympathetic to expanding the PA role and much more negative about expanding the NP role because they can be viewed as more direct competition. So the doctors tend to squelch it through their influence on the Medical Practice Act. I suspect there is a similar story in almost every state.

FREMD: Nationally, there is a trend to try to restrict non-M.D. practice through the Medical Practice Act; however, there have not been attempts in California as yet. I can tell you that in California most doctors are very happy to work alongside NPs and PAs in a wide variety of settings.

The patient safety issue is something that is brought out during testimony for every scope-of-practice expansion effort, not just those involving nurse practitioners. However, all of the research data show that NPs are as safe as doctors when performing the same services. PA and certified-nurse-midwife studies have similar outcomes on patient safety when compared to a physician cohort. So although raising safety concerns may be a good argument from the perspective of physician professional organizations—since the lay public assumes that non-M.D. training must mean less safety—the research doesn't support that. We need to do a better job publicizing the data so the general public will understand.

RS: **Are doctors afraid that the nurses are going out on their own?**
FREMD: Naturally, doctors want to protect their turf and ultimately their income.

In two-thirds of the states, NPs, PAs, and certified nurse-midwives have some level of supervision by physicians, while in the remaining third they do not. These states, including Washington and Arizona, are deemed to have true "independent practice." Although the scope-of-practice language varies in these states, it permits NPs to practice to the fullest extent of their educational preparation and clinical competency. This includes prescriptive authority without supervision oversight.

PAs always practice under some form of physician supervision. Whether the physician needs to be in the office during the patient visit varies from state to state. In California, the doctor does not have to be present.

RS: **Do NPs and PAs differ on policy issues?**
FREMD: NPs and PAs often work together on policy issues; the degree and frequency varies from state to state. Improving access to health care services, especially in rural and metro areas, is the main legislative focus in the coming years. In California, the NP and PA organizations have worked on eight bills together and supported dozens of others. They concern changes in prescriptive authority, signing for medication samples, supervision of medical assistants, determination of disability status, providing informed consent for blood transfusions, and other matters.

RS: **How do you see the next few years in California in terms of NPs and PAs, and what will be the impact on physician supply?**
FREMD: California is currently leading a major health care reform initiative to

improve access to health care services, and NPs and PAs (and certified nurse-midwives) are included in that model. Numerous studies have demonstrated the lack of physician supply, especially in primary care. A Petris Center report notes that 20 to 30 percent of California's health care needs are currently met by advanced-practice providers, and that number is expected to grow.[16]

CHRONIC CARE MODELS AND TURF BATTLES

GARY GITNICK, M.D., is a professor of medicine and chief of the Division of Digestive Diseases at the UCLA School of Medicine. He heads the largest gastroenterology division in the world. He was chief of staff of the UCLA Medical Center and was medical director of the UCLA Health Care Programs. He was president of the Medical Board of California, and founded the Fulfillment Fund, which provides long-term educational mentoring to disadvantaged students.

RS: **What is the best way to deliver chronic care—especially to the underserved?**
GITNICK: Chronic care is a massive and expensive problem. Something like 20 percent of the Medicaid dollars are used solely to treat people with diabetes and its complications. Rheumatoid arthritis care is big too.

RS: **Are there promising models that you're seeing to get a handle on this?**
GITNICK: In San Diego County there is an effort called Project Dolce, which uses a population-based delivery system that includes everyone who is on some form of indigent care. You hook them to a TV monitor and follow their blood sugar and complications, and so on. One physician can monitor all these patients via a group of TVs in a room. He then directs treatment by communicating by email or telemedicine with physician assistants and primary care doctors throughout the county.

> *One physician can monitor all these patients via a group of TVs in a room.*

The great thing about this model is that it provides a higher level of care to indigent people, and at the same time it's very cost-effective. And it includes the doctor on the front line, which not all chronic care models do.

RS: **How is the California Medical Board addressing the role of NPs and PAs in the state?**
GITNICK: We try to look at what we think is safe, but there's very little in the way of hard data on that. The board, unlike prior medical boards, is exceptionally consumer-oriented, rather than being essentially a trade organization protecting the doctors.

RS: What happens with bills about scope of practice when the nursing side overlaps with procedures that only doctors had been doing previously. How does that get resolved?

GITNICK: We may step in and oppose the bill. Every health care bill going through committee comes to us for our review. If the nurses want a change to the Medical Practice Act, they have to propose an amendment. Then, if we think it would impinge on patient safety, we and the California Medical Association would strongly oppose it.

RS: How does the Board feel about NPs and PAs writing prescriptions?

GITNICK: We would pretty much oppose anyone writing a drug prescription except under a doctor's supervision. Whether the doctor has to be in the same building or just available by phone is something under active discussion now. We think it has to be a supervisory role, not just a consultation role.

RS: But other types of medical triage go on all the time. You might have a patient in trouble and you can't help them yourself so you send them on to the next level of care. Why can't the standard be, hypothetically, that the NP or PA knows to alert the doctor? Isn't that the way medical practice happens anyhow?

Why can't the standard be, hypothetically, that the NP or PA knows to alert the doctor? Isn't that the way medical practice happens anyhow? [RS]

GITNICK: Yes, but you have to be able to recognize that the problem exists.

RS: I certainly agree there's a difference between recognizing and treating a problem. I can recognize when my car has a flat tire, but I can't fix the damn thing. I call in AAA.

FREE MEDICAL EDUCATION—WITH STRINGS

DONALD GOLDMANN, M.D., is senior vice president of the Institute for Healthcare Improvement (IHI). He is on the infectious diseases clinical staff at Children's Hospital Boston, and he is a professor of pediatrics at Harvard Medical School and a professor of immunology and infectious diseases at the Harvard School of Public Health. His research group applies the principles of clinical epidemiology to the study of clinical outcomes of nosocomial infections.

RS: **What do you think of the potential of the medical home notion?**
GOLDMANN: It is a promising concept for improving coordination of care. However, it will not work if we merely ask physicians to do more work. They already are overtaxed. Rather, we need to create health care teams that work with patients and families to develop a shared care plan. Nurses and other health professionals will need to work together with primary care physicians. Of course, reimbursement mechanisms will have to recognize the roles of all of the members of these care teams. Information technology will play a major role.

RS: **Is there anybody working on ways to make care efficient?**
GOLDMANN: Actually, the best examples I know of are from nursing. One of our projects is called the Transforming Care at the Bedside Project that we're doing with funding from the Robert Wood Johnson Foundation. This is a sixteen-institution prototyping study looking at ways to improve nursing retention, satisfaction, and productivity. The measure is time at the bedside. They found that something like 70 percent of nursing time was spent in non-bedside tasks—administrative work, hunting and gathering, meetings, and so forth. So by redefining what they do and smoothing the system so that things are where they're supposed to be, they've actually reversed that ratio. Now the majority of time is spent at the bedside in most of those institutions.

RS: **Have you got an example that relates directly to physicians?**
GOLDMANN: In physician office practice there is the issue of face-to-face appointments with patients who really don't need that. Frequently what makes it worse is that the patient's problem hasn't been articulated in advance, the consultant's report isn't there, the staff hasn't told the doctor what the patient needs in the way of prevention. If those things aren't teed up for the face-to-face visits, most of them are wasted. So it's important to change the incentives

so that it's more about how you use technology and virtual visits and asynchronous communication to do things that would have required a doctor before.

RS: Another thing I hear about a lot from physician practices is that their productivity is really limited by having to deal with managed care companies. Is that how you see it?

GOLDMANN: Absolutely. The payers all want to have influence on physician practice so that it's more evidence-based. Any given practice has three, five, seven different payers, all of them sending reminders that say things like, "This is what your diabetes patients ought to be getting and are not getting." But it's all a little different, and it comes from seven separate sources. Then when it comes time to deal with the paperwork to try and satisfy the multiple payers, everybody's running around like idiots. Fortunately, the CMS created codes so at least the billing would capture processes for which they were going to be paid. But it's still a nightmare. In this country, a lot of this is still not computerized.

> *Any given practice has three, five, seven different payers, all of them sending reminders that say things like, "This is what your diabetes patients ought to be getting and are not getting."*

RS: At the same time, a lot of our doctors are struggling with an enormous educational debt. What can we do about that?

GOLDMANN: If it were up to me, I'd make medical school free.

RS: They essentially do that in the U.K. and Western Europe. And afterward, the doctors are really civil servants. For example, in Italy, it used to be easy to get into medical school. There were plenty of slots. But afterward, you had to compete for a job because the government was pretty much the only source of employment for physicians. So if you couldn't get a job with the government, you drove a taxi cab.

GOLDMANN: That's the downside. I just know that we have the ability to make it less expensive up front rather than the way it is now.

RS: Right, the American model lets you do what you want and practice wherever you want. In the British system there's a list of vacancies for you to choose from. Of course, the primary care doctors are overpaid right now because some incentives and targets for them were set too low. In any case, you're the first person I've talked to about this who recommends making medical school free. We don't make law school free or dental school free or any of the professional schools. It would just be unprecedented to do that.

GOLDMANN: Maybe so, but I won't give money to Harvard until they make medical school tuition free for anybody who could otherwise not afford it.

> *I won't give money to Harvard until they make medical school tuition free for anybody who could otherwise not afford it.*

RS: Well, luckily, Harvard doesn't need your money. What do you think of the Florida model, which is more geared to the needs of the community and not attached to teaching hospitals?[17] It's much less expensive to do it this way.

GOLDMANN: It makes it more of a trade school that prepares people for what they're going to do. I like that idea.

RS: Do we need to step up training?

GOLDMANN: Opening new medical schools, as opposed to totally reorienting the way in which we train doctors for multidisciplinary care, seems to me to be a very simplistic solution. I am intrigued by Elliott Fisher's data showing that wherever there's more supply, there's more use and not higher quality.[18] I'm very concerned about the fall in primary care doctors, but I don't think training people for a broken system is going to keep them in the system. The incentives aren't lined up.

RS: I agree. We still train doctors to practice by themselves, make all their own decisions, and be the master of their fate.

GOLDMANN: Right, we have to reset expectations. There are a lot of things that doctors do that are deeply satisfying. Today somehow I found a half hour to sit with a dying woman who has an infection-related issue that I know a whole lot about, as well as its context. Without getting maudlin about it, I have a breadth of knowledge and experience to bring to that bedside that no nurse or primary care doctor could. That is always going to be an important part of medicine.

I don't know of any knowledge coupler or artificial intelligence application that really replaces that ability. But that will erode if we don't provide doctors with the time and the means to cultivate those skills, as opposed to all the useless things they have to do 90 percent of the time.

UNDERSTANDING THE REAL COST
OF MEDICAL EDUCATION

ATUL GROVER, M.D., PH.D., is associate director of the Center for Workforce Studies at the Association of American Medical Colleges. He lectures and conducts workshops for leaders in academic medicine. He is a board-certified internist and practicing hospitalist with a doctorate in health and public policy. Earlier, he served as chief medical officer in the National Center for Health Workforce Analysis at the Health Resources and Services Administration.

RS: **What do you think of my $1 million estimate of the cost to train a doctor?**

GROVER: The average figure might be right, but the specialties are different. Some are probably a net zero proposition. If you talk to hospital administrators, they'll tell you, "My family practice is a loss leader service." So their whole enterprise in general internal medicine and family practice might be losing money.

> *If you talk to hospital administrators, they'll tell you, "My family practice is a loss leader service."*

RS: **What about other specialties?**

GROVER: If you're looking at an interventional cardiology trainee who's had three years of internal medicine and then a three- or four-year fellowship in cardiology, he may be making money for the hospital by the end of training. I don't think you can say the same for pediatric rheumatologists. They're not making money because of the patients they see. That's where the economics of the issue become pretty complicated to sort out.

RS: **The Institute of Medicine tried that about thirty or forty years ago and had people fill out time and motion studies, and little forms about how you spend your time. That was a joke. The point I'm making is that whether the total cost of medical education is $1 million or $2 million, it's a lot. And the more specialized you are in the higher-reimbursement specialties, the lower the cost is. I make an estimate that the cost of training a doctor is about $1 million.**

GROVER: That's probably a reasonable assumption.

RS: **What part of GME would you include as the cost of training a doctor?**
GROVER: I would only include the direct side, the DME. If you go back to
the legislation, it essentially says that indirect medical education (IME) is a
proxy for all the other activities that are important in teaching hospitals, and
they couldn't find a way to quantify them. They said, "Well, it looks like this
resident-to-bed ratio correlates pretty well with the amount of research that
they're doing, and the amount of care for the underserved, and with the case
mix index that we might not pick up with our traditional measures." So I really would hold them separately from the DME payments.

RS: **Should we build new medical schools?**
GROVER: Yes. We're up to 17,400 matriculants in the last class, and the projections from the latest surveys of current medical school deans, coupled with
the information we have about new medical schools, suggests that we're
probably on track right now to expand by about 18 percent by the year 2012.
So we're getting closer.

RS: **Of course the bottleneck is on the GME side.**
GROVER: Right. We managed to expand GME a lot in the years following
the implementation of the prospective payment system because it really did
make the payments for GME explicit. That growth plateaued in 1993 and
1994 when you saw inpatient utilization go down as a result of managed care
and the attempt to move more care to the outpatient setting.

We tend to blame the lack of GME growth on the Balanced Budget Act
of 1997, but in fact, that plateau really happened a few years before that. So
I think we won't see the kind of growth that we need—commensurate with
the growth in undergraduate medical education—until we have some kind of
relief from those caps on payment. It's particularly bad in California.

RS: **What will be the impact of nurse practitioners and physician assistants
relative to the physician supply in the coming years?**
GROVER: As a nation, we're slowly learning that we can develop and deliver
services in ways that don't necessarily require physicians, and that's a good
thing. I think NPs and PAs will continue to expand their scope of practice,
and they'll continue to work in every specialty and every setting. The major

limiting factor is going to be their educational infrastructure. I don't see them producing more than another 150,000 or 160,000 NPs and PAs over the next two decades.

RS: **It's a problem. In California there are five bills that would increase the scope of practice of NPs and PAs, mostly on the prescription drug side.**
GROVER: Some individual practices like Greenfield Clinic in Oregon are doing a great job using people efficiently and effectively. I think that most of the real benefits are going to be not from what we can provide through NPs and PAs but through our use of lower-level providers like RNs, CNAs, and medical assistants.

RS: **Do we have a physician shortage?**

I'd say that we probably are at equilibrium, but there's an incredibly severe maldistribution.

GROVER: Right now, I'd say that we probably are at equilibrium, but there's an incredibly severe maldistribution. In California there will be a shortage, but not as great as in some other parts of the country. Given the lack of infrastructure for medical education, I think it's going to be a constant struggle to attract doctors to California once national shortages put a little more pressure on the marketplace.

The shortage is going to be worse for patients and populations that are already underserved. In parts of New York City and San Francisco and Los Angeles we're not going to have a problem. But I think we'll see shortages in the Midwest and in rural and inner-city, and underserved areas.

PRIMARY CARE: HOW MUCH DOES MONEY MATTER?

KEVIN GRUMBACH, M.D., is professor and chair of family and community medicine at the University of California, San Francisco and chief of family and community medicine at San Francisco General Hospital. He is the director of the UCSF Center for California Health Workforce Studies. He coauthored *Understanding Health Policy: A Clinical Approach*, which was excerpted in serial form by the *Journal of the American Medical Association.*

RS: **Does subsidizing GME pay off for the U.S.?**
GRUMBACH: I'm a believer that there should be public investment in medical education, but I think you can't have it the way it is now, with no accountability for the dollars that are invested. So I'd go the other way: there should be continued substantial investment, but linked to much more explicit workforce policy and goals.

RS: **We don't have any workforce policy.**
GRUMBACH: That's the problem. You get $8 or $9 billion a year in Medicare GME with not many strings attached. It's not structured right. The hospitals don't want to pay for ambulatory care-focused training. You'd have to have some way of supporting primary care. Frankly, they should take it out of the hospital-based training and create general practice residencies funded through a separate mechanism.

RS: **Why is there declining interest in primary care?**
GRUMBACH: I think it's the signals that students are getting about what's going to make for a satisfying career, and money counts. The whole lifestyle and the work demands are the other part of that, but I have stopped falling on my sword in terms of our failure in medical education institutions. More and more students are coming out $100,000, $200,000 in debt, and if they see an income potential of $150,000 versus $400,000, frankly, that's going to sway them. On top of that, the higher-paid specialties often come with a less demanding schedule, less uncertainty, more shift work, and more control over your life generally. So my interpretation of the primary care surge in the mid-1990s wasn't because the schools suddenly did something different. I

think the students were getting signals that managed care was going to reduce the number of jobs in specialty care.

RS: Can nurse practitioners and physician assistants fill in the gap in primary care?

GRUMBACH: When you start looking at the hourly fee, NPs and PAs are not such a bargain anymore. And there are different expectations about overtime arrangements and whether they'll take on-call. The nonphysicians are most likely going to give you thirty-five or forty hours, not the fifty or sixty you often get from doctors. The fact is that they are bailing out of primary care just like the physicians. I think hospitals are increasingly hiring them, because of the work hours reductions for residents. We have trauma nurse practitioners now in San Francisco General.

When you start looking at the hourly fee, NPs and PAs are not such a bargain anymore.

But in primary care now it's all about the medical assistants. That's where the action is. There aren't many RNs working in ambulatory or primary care. Again, they're too expensive there.

RS: They're pooled in the hospital?

GRUMBACH: Right, so the mainstays in most primary care offices are the medical assistants; maybe some LVNs and LPNs. The few RNs who work there are usually doing major case-management-type work. In fact, I'm really intrigued by the wonderful, innovative models we're seeing out there with a lot of the chronic care and preventive care delegated out. These are very protocol-driven types of care, so the challenge is to make it more automated and routinized. The staff can be flagged when diabetic patients are due for a foot exam. The physician doesn't have to flip through charts or even electronic medical records to find out when somebody needs a mammogram.

RS: The doctors would be doing what they were trained to do.

GRUMBACH: Exactly. That's why I like a lean supply configuration—it forces you to be more creative and deploy people at a maximum level of skill.

A REGIONAL APPROACH TO HEALTH DISPARITIES

RISA LAVIZZO-MOUREY, M.D., is president and CEO of the Robert Wood Johnson Foundation. She was director of the Institute on Aging, University of Pennsylvania, and chief of the Division of Geriatric Medicine. She served in the U.S. Department of Health and Human Services as deputy administrator of the Agency for Health Care Research and Quality. Dr. Lavizzo-Mourey was a member of the White House Task Force on Health Care Reform and was a consultant to the White House on issues of health policy.

RS: **What will it take to improve provider performance in chronic care?**
LAVIZZO-MOUREY: A lot of studies suggest that the quality of care is not nearly what it should be, given that we pay more than any other country in the world. We're not at the top of the heap on many health indicators. To improve the quality of care, everyone who has a stake in it will have to work together, and I think that is going to have to be done at a regional level.

RS: **Why the regional level?**
LAVIZZO-MOUREY: First you absolutely need to have national standards and guidelines in order to improve the quality of care. But then you've got to have people working together in a more local environment to measure what they do, see how they stand relative to the national standards, dive deeply into ways they aren't measuring up, and come up with plans to improve.

RS: **What would it take to get from here to there?**
LAVIZZO-MOUREY: It will take some regional commitment on the part of health care providers, employers, patients, and individual physician practices. That's not going to be done without a strong commitment to measurement and to transparency. It will take a big investment in information systems so that this kind of reporting can be done much more simply. And of course there will have to be some change in the payment system.

RS: **Will pay for performance help get us there? Medicare recently announced that it will no longer pay for so-called "avoidable errors." That's an important statement.**
LAVIZZO-MOUREY: Yes. The fact that CMS is making bold changes to align the incentives better with high-quality care is just one of the steps that will have

to happen. It is going to require ever-increasing measurement of outcomes and then rewarding people with a variety of mechanisms. Financial payments are one kind of reward, but there are others, like incentives to have a more sophisticated information system, for example.

RS: **There is a problem of disparities in Americans' access to health care—in part along socioeconomic and racial or ethnic lines. Would greater access to health insurance ameliorate this problem?**

LAVIZZO-MOUREY: Well, there is evidence that when people get Medicare coverage there's some decrease in the disparity across racial and ethnic groups in terms of health care services used. So you can make the argument that if we could give people insurance, there would likely be a decrease in disparities related to access. But that's not the same as reducing disparities in terms of health status, life expectancy, or infant mortality, where a lot of other factors come into play.

RS: **Aside from the political and financial challenges to providing broad insurance coverage, there are the supply-side issues, as economists like to call them. In a nutshell, the problem is that if everyone in the country suddenly had appropriate, speedy access to care, there would be massive new demands on the system.**

The problem is that if everyone in the country suddenly had appropriate, speedy access to care, there would be massive new demands on the system. [RS]

LAVIZZO-MOUREY: Well, anything we do to ensure that people have health insurance is not likely to happen overnight. It is going to be a multiyear process. But if we could provide insurance coverage to everyone, we would have to offer services in ways that are not limited to what individual physicians do now. For example, there are experiments in which care is being delivered in pharmacies, in schools, and in a growing number of outpatient surgical clinics. In fact, there are lots of different avenues that could be augmented in order to meet the demand of the mainly pre-Medicare population that would newly be covered by insurance.

RS: **There's been an issue for a long time in the health care workforce about what is sometimes called ethnic concordance. In California, for example,** we're within a few years of being a predominantly Hispanic state, but the number of Hispanic doctors is only around 5 to 6 percent. At the same time, doctors of Asian ancestry are overrepresented in comparison to the population. And the proportion of African-American physicians is decreasing. Should the ethnicity of the doctor workforce roughly mirror that of a given population?

LAVIZZO-MOUREY: There's good evidence that people are more satisfied and more likely to listen to the advice of a provider they trust; and the level of trust between patients and providers where there is concordance has been shown in the literature to be higher. Data suggest that among certain specialties, there isn't adequate diversity. Some people are not referred for renal transplantation or for certain types of lung cancer surgery at an early stage because there's not a trusted specialist to receive that referral.

Data suggest that among certain specialties, there isn't adequate diversity.

RS: So is concordance an appropriate goal?

LAVIZZO-MOUREY: I would look deeper than that. If you have a system for producing physicians that is fair and equitable, then a particular ethnic group in the population *would* be represented among the professionals in that area. If it's not, then you have to ask yourself, "Why is there a discordance?"

A SHORT HISTORY OF MEDICAL EDUCATION AND DIVERSITY

PHILIP R. LEE, M.D., is senior scholar, Institute for Health Policy Studies, and professor emeritus of social medicine at the University of California, San Francisco. He is a consulting professor in human biology at Stanford University. From 1993 to 1997, Dr. Lee served as assistant secretary for health, U.S. Department of Health and Human Services. He was a founder and director of the Institute for Health Policy Studies, and served as chancellor of UCSF. He was Assistant Secretary for Health and Scientific Affairs in the Department of Health, Education, and Welfare from 1965 to 1969.

RS: Tell me about the early days in medical education at UCSF.

LEE: During the period from 1963, and particularly after the Civil Rights Act, which began to impact medical education in the late 1960s, you saw a very dramatic shift in admissions to medical schools. Of course, Howard and Meharry—predominantly black schools—lost some of their best applicants to Harvard, Yale, Stanford, UCSF, and a variety of other schools. The numbers of minorities in medical schools increased significantly, as did the percentage, until the Supreme Court's Bakke decision in 1978 forbade the use of racial quotas.

At that point, there was also a shift in policy. The federal government started focusing on the problems of geographic and specialty maldistribution. Along the way, their attitude toward medical education shifted from seeing it as a public good to a market good. Charlie Edwards,[19] in testimony in the mid-1970s, actually said the medical students should pay for their own education, because they're going to make a lot of money as practitioners. In other words, it was no longer the community's responsibility to ensure an adequate physician supply for the population. It was more the individual's responsibility.

RS: That certainly didn't work to the benefit of minorities in medicine.

LEE: No, not until the early 1990s, when there was, again, a movement among medical schools to increase the number of minorities. At that time the Association of American Medical Colleges (AAMC) was in a leadership position. That was short-lived, particularly after California voters amended the state constitution to prohibit public institutions from discriminating on the basis of race, sex, or ethnicity. It only affected the University of California, but

Texas, Florida, Washington, and a number of other states took anti-affirmative action policies at the state level.

RS: **I remember that you did a lot at UCSF for minorities, particularly in primary care.**
LEE: Well, they say it's a good idea to ride the horse in the direction it's going. A small group of leaders had gotten things started in the early 1960s. The goal was to have 25 percent underrepresented minorities by the end of the decade. There were a number of Jewish faculty, who remembered quotas when they were going to school, and they absolutely did not want a quota. We achieved the goal, but it was a very different approach. It was rooted first in a group of faculty. Then, after Martin Luther King's assassination, it was rooted in the black caucus and the black student union, which played a very significant role in stimulating the campus.

RS: **What was the climate like there while this was going on?**
LEE: The campus, at that point, Richard, would be hard to describe. There was segregation. If you were a black college graduate and you had served in the Navy, and you had run a laboratory, the only job you could get would be as a janitor. At UCSF they had to eat their meals in the basement. One of the black faculty members said to me, "Phil, you know what we call UCSF? We call it the plantation." So that was the climate.

RS: **Keeping that history in mind, what should we be trying to achieve now? If there are x number of African-Americans in the population, and y number of Latinos, ought there to be some corresponding portion of black and Latino doctors in the community?**
LEE: A lot of people think so, but I wouldn't agree with that. In California, there's been a big influx of Latino population, but a lot of the minority doctors are coming from the Asian community.

The biggest change has been the increase in women medical students. Among African-Americans, there are significant numbers of women—more women than men. That's also true among Asians, although the numbers are more equal.

> *The biggest change has been the increase in women medical students. Among African-Americans, there are more women than men.*

RS: **Why should we try to have minorities in medical school? Why is this worth fighting for?**

LEE: Well, first, it enhances the education of all the students. We see that very significantly at Stanford with the undergraduates. They have a very diverse student body and a strong program of student financial aid. No student gets barred for financial reasons. Since Stanford is a private university, there is no anti-affirmative action policy like there is at public institutions.

Another reason for diversity is that young people ought to have the opportunity to go to medical school. We argued about the insufficient number of places in the medical schools in the 1960s. A lot of legislators wanted to increase enrollment so kids from their districts could go to medical school.

RS: **And it's also true that being a doctor is a high-status, highly paid occupation. So there is the issue of giving minorities access to that, which is different from saying that they will be delivering medical care, perhaps, to their corresponding minority populations.**

LEE: Yes, and they do treat minority populations more. And it's also true that people of different backgrounds like to have doctors who understand their culture, speak their language. In the recent hiring at the Palo Alto Clinic, we had ten doctors. One was male, an anesthesiologist. The other nine were women— all in family medicine or general internal medicine. All of them spoke English, and more than half spoke Spanish as well. A third of them spoke Mandarin. One spoke Serbo-Croatian. Another one spoke Taiwanese, and another Tagalog.

Since the 1980s, I have tried to promote the idea of sending U.S. doctors and students to practice in other countries where they are needed. We've got a handful of doctors who work overseas, and they do good stuff.

RS: **Do you think residency programs could be induced to send some of their students abroad?**

LEE: Actually, many undergraduate students do that already, and they love it. I think at the residency level it would be a very, very valuable experience. It could be a six-month or a one-year rotation, let's say, in a hospital in a country where they could get excellent training, but where there aren't enough doctors. A lot of our medical schools—UCSF, Washington, and Stanford, that I know of directly—have major AIDS programs. They could incorporate a lot of the medical school's learning in the overseas programs.

TOO MANY DOCTORS, TOO LITTLE EFFICIENCY

ARNOLD MILSTEIN, M.D., is medical director at the Pacific Business Group on Health and the National Health Care Thought Leader at William M. Mercer. He worked with the National Committee for Quality Assurance (NCQA) to develop the Healthcare Effectiveness Data and Information Set (HEDIS), and is a member of the Performance Measures Coordinating Committee. Dr. Milstein is an associate clinical professor at the University of California, San Francisco Medical Center, and an elected member of the Institute of Medicine.

RS: What is the best way to address a doctor shortage? Camp 1 says we should get doctors we already have to work smarter, better, more efficiently. Camp 2 wants to train more doctors and get them out there.
MILSTEIN: I'm definitely in Camp 1.

RS: Then you're kind of a rare bird, although some of the economists are with you in Camp 1 just because that's the way economists think. There are a lot of people in Camp 2, and I think that is based on the notion that doctors are rigid; you can get them to change their behavior somewhat—as managed care did—but it's hard to move them dramatically. On the efficiency side, what are some things that can be done with specialists?
MILSTEIN: We should routinize quality-adjusted "contract capitation" payment and concentrate referrals with the most efficient specialists. Contract capitation means a standardized fixed amount for all services associated with the initial phase of a specialist's care. In their diagnostic and initial treatment plans, specialists would become much more mindful of total resources consumed. For ongoing specialist care, quality-adjusted and severity-adjusted monthly capitation would serve the same objective.

RS: You're thinking that economic efficiency is driven by putting this risk back on the specialist.
MILSTEIN: Yes. Before HMOs reduced their risk transfer to physicians, several California managed care medical groups found that capitation substantially lowered the average level of intensity of specialist care without lowering quality scores.

At the same time, we should encourage faster evolution of efficiency-enhancing health professional roles such as hospitalists and lay health coaches. Even in the absence of risk transfer to providers, the hospitalist notion has "stuck" because, in addition to enhancing the overall efficiency of care, it saved attending physicians from driving back and forth to the hospital to visit one or two patients.

> *A good example of efficiency is nurse-run anticoagulation and diabetic wound care clinics.*

Another good example of efficiency is nurse-run anticoagulation and diabetic wound care clinics, which have substantially reduced complications that require expensive physician and hospital intervention. These and similar labor-mix innovations shift interventions to more cost-effective health care workers. They're a by-product of systems thinking.

RS: Do you see a lot of value in the systems approach?

MILSTEIN: Absolutely. For it to flourish, payment incentives have to focus physician and hospital leaders on testing innovations that lower total payer spending and quality defects. For example, (1) modify the fee-for-service payment system via a quality-adjusted virtual capitation; (2) re-set fee-for-service payments so they reflect prices in non-oligopolized provider markets; and (3) introduce a plus-or-minus 20 percent variation from fee-for-service payment based on a provider's rank on quality and on conservation of total payer spending per episode for acute illness and per year for chronic and preventive care.

Virtual capitation is necessary for provider aggregations too small to bear *full* capitation risk. For larger health systems, quality-adjusted actual capitation geared to national benchmark levels of quality and low total population spending would be less complex.

RS: And you profile providers.

MILSTEIN: Exactly. Fee for service, in its current form, encourages useless services. We should give robust incentives to providers to excel in both low total spending and quality. By gradually moving toward a 40 percent variation in payment rates between providers in the highest and lowest deciles, we'd create a "burning platform," while enabling providers reasonable lead time to

> *By gradually moving toward a 40 percent variation in payment rates we'd create a "burning platform."*

master "implementation science." I think the result could be exponential—a health care equivalent of Moore's Law.

RS: **How did you arrive at the percentage?**
MILSTEIN: A 40 percent differential between highest and lowest performers is large enough to offset the 30 percent of service volume that Dartmouth research has demonstrated to be useless. Incentives for efficiency must be larger than 30 percent to wean providers from income based on performing useless services.

RS: **That's a lot. So this national fee schedule is something like a relative value scale or a prospective payment.**
MILSTEIN: Exactly. It's a value-based relative value scale rather than resource-based.

RS: **But I thought you were an outcomes guy.**
MILSTEIN: I am. Both of my targets are outcomes. Total risk-adjusted per person spending is a financial outcome measure. In the near term, quality measures would need to include process measures along with intermediate outcome measures like hemoglobin A1c and surgical complication rates. In the meantime, we should challenge health services researchers to come up with health status change measures that are more widely applicable than the SF-36.

RS: **What about quality measures?**
MILSTEIN: I don't think you need perfect measures to have the desired effect. Look at the evolution in car safety measures. It began with "seat belts: yes or no" and evolved to include very sophisticated safety systems. But we would never have gotten to electronic stability control and eight airbags had we not started with "seat belts: yes or no."

RS: **Right. Whenever we try something like that in the policy world, the side that doesn't want to do it tries to defeat it because it's not perfect.**
MILSTEIN: The health industry is wealthy and politically powerful. However, I believe resistance to performance-based payment and patient referral will eventually be overcome by progressive health industry leaders and middle-class worry about health insurance affordability and quality of care.

RS: Physician profiling tries to get at that. Over time, it will narrow the distribution, push it toward the mean.

MILSTEIN: I hope not. I don't think we should reward movement toward the mean. We should reward movement toward the performance frontier on both total cost of care and quality.

RS: You were involved for years in the Pacific Business Group on Health's report cards on medical group, health plan, and hospital performance. It was administered to patients. There was controversy and even lawsuits around that, but the program didn't really have a lot of teeth.

MILSTEIN: It was a very important predecessor to the P4P and tiered network plans that followed. They continue to rely on similar measurement methods. The seeds we planted helped propel the transparency and value-purchasing movements that are rapidly spreading.

RS: Would it be reasonable to say that the report cards didn't really affect the selection by patients to any large degree? I've always been puzzled by that.

MILSTEIN: As Judy Hibbard and Arnie Epstein showed, they had more impact on providers.[20] It was probably a combination of embarrassment, natural competitiveness, and fear that it would affect patient volume over time. What matters is that providers worry it will have an effect.

These worries are coming to fruition via the current spread of tiered network benefit plans. They're like tiered formularies; the amount the consumer pays is linked to the quality and efficiency rating of the doctor or hospital they select. It's unfolding in more than a hundred markets.

RS: So if I want better quality and efficiency, I pay more?

MILSTEIN: Exactly the opposite. If you select a physician or hospital that ranks more favorably, you pay less.

RS: That would drive patients to efficient places, which would then have higher volume. It would also move the rest of the market in the direction of efficiency.

MILSTEIN: Exactly. Meredith Rosenthal and I wrote a paper about tiered network plans being the promising iteration of consumerism.[21] We know that they save money. They've already enabled 3 to 10 percent lower premiums. An important remaining question is whether the lower spending is due to patients staying with the doctors they like and paying more out-of-pocket, or to patients switching to the better performers. I think it depends somewhat on the income level of the enrollees.

RS: **How would capitation work in tiered network plans?**
MILSTEIN: No differently than in nontiered plans. The most favorably tiered providers would be those with the lowest quality-adjusted (actual or virtual) capitation rates.

RS: **The tiered physician network idea operates by the same principle as tiered formularies, except the product that is being tiered is physicians.**
MILSTEIN: Yes. Two variants are becoming prevalent. One tier is based solely on quality, and it is based on adherence to clinical guidelines using claims data. We know from Beth McGlynn's work that the average frequency is about 55 percent.[22] The second tier adds the "total cost of care dimension." Episode-grouping software captures all costs associated with an episode of acute care or with a year of chronic and preventive care. For each episode or year, attribution algorithms identify the most accountable physician(s) whose risk-adjusted average total spending can be compared to specialty-matched norms.

RS: **As a consumer, then, I would be given choices by my plan. If I go to A, I'm going to pay a certain percent. If I go to B or C, I'm going to pay more. Is that right?**
MILSTEIN: Yes. Consumers would have incentives to select better-rated providers. Another approach is to design the plan so that the consumer pays a lower premium or deductible in exchange for agreeing to use a select group of doctors for non-emergency care. It's a "decision and consequence" approach geared to a single annual decision rather than to many point-of-service decisions during a year. The most prevalent form is variable coinsurance or copay based on point-of-service decisions. We're in an era of experimentation on this, and there's no standardization of either approach. For example, some insurers are creating two provider performance cut points, and therefore three tiers.

RS: **What kind of initial productivity increase could you get? Would it be 5 percent, 10 percent, 20 percent?**

MILSTEIN: Richard, I know this is going to sound crazy, but I think it's more like 50 percent.

RS: **How could that be?**

MILSTEIN: The upside is very large. Look at what Eugene Litvak did with a handful of hospitals by applying a very simple engineering concept like level-scheduling elective admissions.[23] One hospital doubled throughput with existing resources while improving quality. I think we're at the very beginning of understanding what we can accomplish via the use of modern implementation science. It's analogous to the "pre-Ford" stage in the American automobile industry, when cars were made in small garages all across the country and operations engineering methods were largely absent. When the change came, it was immense.

The current period is analogous to the "pre-Ford" stage in the American automobile industry, when cars were made in small garages all across the country. When the change came, it was immense.

RS: **What period of time are you talking about for health care productivity to shoot up?**

MILSTEIN: Ten years after (1) we create a profoundly performance-sensitive environment around doctors and hospitals, and (2) interoperable clinical information systems adoption exceeds 90 percent.

TAKING RESPONSIBILITY FOR GENERATING AMERICA'S DOCTORS

FITZHUGH MULLAN, M.D., is a pediatrician and the Murdock Head Professor of Medicine and Health Policy in the George Washington University's School of Public Health and Health Services. He is a contributing editor to *Health Affairs* and the editor of that journal's "Narrative Matters" section. Dr. Mullan is director of the Hirsh Program in Medicine and Public Policy.

RS: **Will the increase in nurse practitioners and physician assistants substantially satisfy the growing demand for care?**

MULLAN: They're a terrific asset, and I think they are exactly the swing factor that we need. The demand is going to go up, and there's going to be stress on the system. But the way you cope with that, quite apart from major structural changes in reimbursement, is the training and deployment of a large, growing, and flexible force of nonphysician clinicians, particularly nurse practitioners and physician assistants.

RS: **Why do you feel that NPs and PAs will be such an important part of the workforce?**

MULLAN: The notion that these are simply primary care helpmates is belied by the marketplace. My mother sees a PA when she goes to her cardiologist. This is a highly skilled person who has been trained in a specific aspect of medical care, and does a good deal of the work of the cardiologist. You also have folks in orthopedics who do much of the ambulatory work in that specialty.

My mother sees a PA when she goes to her cardiologist. This is a highly skilled person who does a good deal of the work of the cardiologist.

The reality is that the physician workforce, on both the primary care side and the specialty side, can be augmented and can be flexible. We're going to see more areas—as in thoracic surgery, where the CABG goes into senescence because it's been replaced by a better technology that doesn't require the cardiac surgeon. If you train everybody to be a cardiac surgeon, you're going to have a bunch of Edsels sitting out in the garage, hardly driven. Having a more flexible base force, like NPs and PAs, I think is the way to build a workforce for the future.

RS: **Do you think we should train more doctors?**

MULLAN: Well, we could train five thousand more physicians per year at the medical school level, and we would still be slightly short of self-sufficient. Right now, between medicine and osteopathy, we graduate about seventeen to eighteen thousand people to take twenty-four thousand PCY1 (residency) positions. So about six thousand are filled by international medical graduates. If we simply train more undergraduates, say nineteen to twenty-two thousand, we would diminish the call on the rest of the world. That would be the outcome I would push for. But the Council of Graduate Medical Education (COGME) and the Association of American of Medical Colleges (AAMC) are calling for an increase in the PGY1 residency slots in the range of thirty thousand so that we can accommodate increasing numbers of U.S. graduates while maintaining or perhaps increasing the draw on the rest of the world.

RS: **What would happen if we did that?**

MULLAN: If you put more doctors out into the workforce, the current ratio of 280 per 100,000 population would gradually become 290, 300, 330, 350. I don't think we should go there. That would send us further down the path of an enormously expensive, fragmented, and specialty-heavy physician workforce.

I think it's a semi-fiction that hospitals need federal support in order to train more residents, but if they do, Medicare's got other things to do with their money.

In any case, I think it's a semi-fiction that hospitals need federal support in order to train more residents, but if they do, Medicare's got other things to do with their money. They shouldn't be pouring it out at $80,000 per resident per year. That's just not a good investment of taxpayers' money.

RS: **What changes would you suggest?**

MULLAN: I would provide incentives and encouragement to medical schools to increase their size. And I think the 280 physicians per 100,000 population may float up to 300. We need to increase the Medicare residency funding cap a little bit because the population is growing 1 percent a year. But I'd keep the cap there. If a hospital wanted more plastic surgeons, say, it could train them "off cap"—add another position but not expect a subsidy for it.

I'm for increasing the medical schools because I think we ought to take responsibility for generating our own doctors. They're out there.

RS: **In fact, about 25 percent of our physicians in practice were trained abroad. A large number of them stay here for their whole career.**
MULLAN: The IMG story goes back to the 1930s and 1940s. It's grown steadily, but stabilized from the mid-1990s on. They take exactly the same exams as U.S. medical graduates, which I feel is a reasonable safety guarantee. These are some of the brightest, most ambitious, and capable people in their countries, and having them here is a huge benefit to the U.S. for that reason.

RS: **What would you say is the downside to that?**
MULLAN: Well, it has blunted the market for U.S. medical school growth because there has been little pressure to educate more U.S. physicians when the world continuously supplies them. That translates into lost opportunity for U.S. students. The barrier for getting into medical school remains very high, and so lots of folks don't make it. Some go to the Caribbean for training, and some give up and go into business or whatever.

RS: **On the other hand, the IMGs are more willing to practice in underserved areas and maybe in less attractive specialties that the U.S. needs. The COGME notion was to pay for 50 percent primary care, 50 percent specialty, and 10 percent more residents than we graduate from U.S. medical schools, not 30 percent more.**
MULLAN: That would have cut the number of international graduates and changed the makeup of the workforce, which is roughly two-thirds specialists, one-third generalist.

RS: **It obviously didn't happen because the market wants specialists; they make more money in the marketplace, and during residency training, the hospitals make more money from their services.**
MULLAN: There's also a question about cultural competency and linguistic ability, which is worth thinking about. One of the ironies is that psychiatry, which is a less sought-after specialty, has become highly attractive to IMGs. Of all the specialties, this must be the most culturally sensitive. So you often

have people with major language barriers trying to communicate with each other over very sensitive personal problems.

RS: **Nevertheless, a lot of people say that having IMGs is a good deal for the U.S. They are educated at the expense of foreign countries, then save us some more money during their residencies as well.**
MULLAN: Taking that rationale to the absurd, we ought to get *all* our health care workers from overseas. Offshore the entire enterprise! What I'm basically saying is that we ought to be self-sufficient in professions in which our country has a wellhead of interest. It's not as if Americans don't want to sign up.

RS: **In a global market, surely people have a right to move where they want.**
MULLAN: Yes, but having calibrated our market the way we have (and Britain and Canada have done similarly) there is a huge vacuum that sucks people out of other countries. We could strip the world bare of nurses. We could strip certain countries close to bare of physicians.

> *We could strip the world bare of nurses. We could strip certain countries close to bare of physicians.*

They don't all come out of Africa, but you don't have to take too many out of Africa to cripple their health systems. We also import physicians from Canada and the U.K. in large numbers to fill our vacuum. Those countries then turn to India, Africa, and the Caribbean to back-fill the doctors they have lost to us. Between the three of us, we take thousands of physicians away from the developing world, destabilizing health systems all over the world. Now you'll be quickly told that there are benefits. On the other hand, if a country is trying to take on HIV . . .

RS: **Do you think the IMGs would be working on those problems if they stayed in their home countries, or would they be involved in high-end medicine?**
MULLAN: Most of the developing countries who are most severely hurt have very, very small markets for high-end practice. To be sure, many of their medical schools train to Western standards. Everybody wants to be the Harvard of wherever. I don't mean that disparagingly, but the standards are distorted by the kind of high-end technology that they see in the West. The health sector

opportunities in most developing countries are predominantly in the public sector. The public health system *is* the system. In the capital you will have a very small elite market that treats the wealthy with as much technology as they can muster, and often the medical school is linked to that culture. But the country doesn't have the ability to absorb the kinds of doctors who are being trained to the Western standards, and it creates a kind of dissonance.

As long as we're taking large percentages of their workforce to the West, these countries are on a rat's wheel. They keep running and they don't get anywhere, and that means people are dying because we're failing to train enough doctors for our own needs.

RS: It's a moral outrage. I hear you loud and clear.

WE EXPECT TOO MUCH FROM PHYSICIANS

EDWARD O'NEIL, PH.D., is a professor in the Departments of Family and Community Medicine, Preventive and Restorative Dental Sciences, and Social and Behavioral Sciences at the University of California, San Francisco. He heads the Center for the Health Professions, a research, advocacy, and training institute. Dr. O'Neil was executive director of the Pew Health Professions Commission, and has been a consultant to the WHO and other major organizations.

RS: **What can you tell me about the cost savings that occurred during the managed care revolution?**
O'NEIL: My reality was that managed care moved in because there was excess bed capacity in hospitals and in physician numbers so that the per diem rates and the reimbursement rates were bid down, and that is really where the cost savings came from. There was some utilization control but it was really the reimbursement rates.

RS: **How did this impact residency slots?**
O'NEIL: Through the late 1980s and early 1990s, when everything was go-go in terms of reimbursement, the number of new residency slots had been increasing by about 10 percent a year. We were filling those partly with osteopaths and increasing numbers of international medical school graduates. As that started to crank down, the government got more stringent on reimbursement and also on approval for new programs. Before that, you would just send in the application, and if you had the ability to do the residency program, then you could hire residents. It was a no-brainer for any hospital administrator. But that went away, and so we stopped growing. Then, with the movement away from primary care reimbursement, we started getting ourselves into the situation we're in today.

RS: **Do medical schools have a sufficiently diverse pool of applicants?**
O'NEIL: From the perspective of the medical school admission committees, the reality is that we could go down two whole standard deviations in the applicant pool and still admit a class that would be successful and far more diverse. Now we wouldn't be dealing with the very best and brightest from every generation, but the reality is that if you're doing family medicine in

some little town, you may not need to be the best and the brightest in your generation. I work a lot with physicians out there in the valley, general practitioners, undifferentiated specialists, general surgeons, ob / gyns, and they are bored out of their minds.

> *If you're doing family medicine in some little town, you may not need to be the best and the brightest in your generation.*

RS: Do we expect too much from physicians?

O'NEIL: You could say that a doctor is this incredibly expensive, million-dollar tool that we're making and we want it to do everything. We want it to manage chronicity in the community, and to do exotic specialty therapeutic care, and sometimes even to differentiate itself into being a biomedical researcher capable of pulling data on RO1 from NIH.[24] And on top of that we want this tool to be bilingual or maybe trilingual. It's just crazy, and it's so emblematic of the whole system, that we've overspecialized and pay way too much money for everything.

It would be better to hire a lot of community health workers for minimum wage plus 50 percent, people who are completely bilingual, people who would actually offer a different level of communication with a patient. The alternative requires that everything be typed out through the hands of the physician, and processed through the mind of the physician. That's ridiculous. It's not just last year's view, it's last century's view.

RS: What do you think the ratio of doctors to population should be?

O'NEIL: At the macro level, we have too often associated health with access to a ratio of physicians to population, and I'm just not sure that pans out. Look at the number of physicians per 100,000 population in Iowa and Connecticut. There's a 100 percent difference—about 140 to over 300—but I can't find any difference in the health of people in Connecticut versus people in Iowa. The only real difference is that health care in Connecticut is much more expensive.

RS: Would training more doctors lead to better quality and cost-effectiveness?

O'NEIL: There's a great experiment that we're living through with the nurse staffing ratios. I haven't seen any dramatic evidence that by increasing those ratios we have changed the quality of care. There is some evidence that we're increasing the cost of care. By the same token I'm not sure that producing more physicians will help in terms of cost or quality. Our health care costs us 16.5 percent of GDP, 100,000 avoidable deaths, and general unhappiness inside and outside the system. In an unkind moment, I have been known to say, "If the beast is not serving you any longer, why would you want to continue feeding it by producing more physicians?"

I have been known to say, "If the beast is not serving you any longer, why would you want to continue feeding it by producing more physicians?"

Rather than build a new medical school in Riverside, the best thing for California to do would be to subsidize the construction of a quasi-public-private osteopathic medical school. It costs a fraction of what an allopathic school does. And a significant proportion of the osteopathic school graduates go on to allopathic residencies, and they are much more likely to go into primary care.[25]

And if we develop shortages in primary care, we can ramp up the production of nurse practitioners. It's expensive to educate young physicians. We need some, but we shouldn't buy all of these very expensive Mercedes if what we are going to need is some basic transportation.

THE INTEGRATED SYSTEM:
PAYING FOR PRIMARY CARE

ROBERT PEARL, M.D., is executive director and CEO of The Permanente Medical Group, headquartered in Oakland, California. He is board-certified in plastic and reconstructive surgery, and he serves on the faculty of the Stanford Medical School, where he is a clinical professor of plastic surgery. Over the past several years, he served as a visiting professor at Stanford Business School, Duke University School of Medicine, and Harvard School of Public Health.

RS: How important is it to match doctors and patients in terms of language, and how do you do this at Kaiser?

PEARL: It's possible to deliver good care through translators, but I have strong feelings that language is a major part of high-quality care. At Kaiser we have very strong programs around providing language adequacy for our members. The days are over when you have to bring your seven-year-old child to translate for the parent; that's just wrong. At the very least, you need a fully trained translator. It's much more efficient to deliver care in a language that you speak, rather than go through the multiple steps of translation with all the risks of miscommunication.

Beyond language, we need to have a level of cultural alignment. With more than six thousand physicians in our organization, we can do that. We try to estimate the demand, and then we listen to what our patients are telling us. All members are asked to select a primary care physician, and within that process, they can express a lot of preferences.

RS: My colleagues and I recently published a paper looking at the salaries of different doctors by their ethnicity, then matching that with the ethnicity of their communities. The findings showed that a minority doctor makes more money in an area where there's less matching of his or her particular ethnicity.[26]

PEARL: So that tells you patients actually value that choice and are willing to pay more for it. I think there is a segment of each population for whom that's a high priority, and another segment for whom it's not.

RS: I suspect the language issue is more important in primary care, because if patients have good communication with the primary care doctor, obviously they can get the right specialty care as well. Would you agree with that?

PEARL: The answer is yes and no. I agree in the sense that with primary care there is a much longer relationship. Our average member spends seventeen years with us. So that's seventeen years' worth of visits, as opposed to their specialist contact.[27]

The other factor is that the number of physicians in specialty departments are usually relatively low, so you don't have the same number of options. We have a thousand primary care physicians to pick among. But if you need a neurosurgeon, there might be twenty. So the ethnicities and the language opportunities are going to be far greater in primary care, and we should be able to provide for almost any preference.

RS: I'm very interested in the use of nurse practitioners and physician assistants. Given that national average salaries (in 2003) were almost $75,000 for NPs and about $80,000 for PAs, are they still an attractive option when the average primary care doctor nationally now makes around $140,000?

PEARL: First of all, we pay primary care doctors dramatically more than that. Whatever the national average salary in primary care is, we're willing to pay more to recruit the top echelon. That said, we've shifted somewhat away from using physician extenders for primary care into specialty care because of the narrower salary difference in primary care than in the past. We've hired a huge number of primary care physicians and reduced the ratio of our patients to physicians by 20 percent over the past three to five years. PAs can't work within primary care because of the contract we have with our nurses union. So historically, all the PAs have worked in specialty care or the emergency room.

RS: Do you think we should educate more physicians, as the AAMC has recommended?

PEARL: I've been a proponent of expanding the number of medical school seats, and I've offered to various local universities to have Kaiser Permanente help lead that process. The residencies are a bit more complex because getting the right number of individuals in each geographic location requires a lot more overall coordination than I think exists in this country. We probably have only half as many doctors going into primary care as we need nationally. Of course, productivity is a big part of the solution.

RS: **What do you do in the Kaiser system to maximize the productivity of doctors?**

PEARL: First, what happens in an integrated system is that you avoid redundancy. So as an example, my dad back East had a melanoma taken off of his nose, and in getting ready for that, he had three histories and physicals and two separate EKGs.

> *What happens in an integrated system is that you avoid redundancy.*

That's typical in a fragmented system. When you're a prepaid system, as opposed to fee for service, you don't have a taxicab mentality that involves a lot of visits that I would say are not only unnecessary, but really inconvenient for patients.

The second thing is the IT system. You can have the EKG done once, and then it's available to everyone online. I think physicians are tired of practicing in the fragmented system of community medicine. They're preferentially going toward places where care is integrated and where they have advanced IT systems to provide them with the data. That's one of the most powerful market changes that has happened.

RS: **I've heard it said that the doctors who work as employees do this mainly to avoid the problems of running their own business.**

PEARL: I'd say that's a misinterpretation. What they really want is to be able to provide the best quality of medical care. That requires a high level of coordination, collaboration, and technology. We have eight physician applicants for every opening; there were more than five thousand applicants last year.

RS: **Do you think Kaiser's emphasis on prevention is part of the attraction?**

PEARL: It is. In fact, we just had a press conference making available to the local communities the approaches that we've used to lower the cardiac mortality for our members 30 percent below that of patients cared for by fee-for-service physicians and community hospitals. A small amount of that improvement has to do with the technical interventions after a heart attack, and creating centers of excellence and consolidating volume for better quality. But a lot of the improvement is simply prevention. As an example, smoking in Northern California has stayed relatively flat and actually has gone up over the past year from 16 percent to 17 percent. We've lowered it for our members to about 9 percent. That's a dramatic difference.

RS: **What do you see as the main problem in health care delivery generally?**
PEARL: You'd never run a business the way American health delivery system is run. Care is fragmented, information technology is limited, and no one oversees capital investment or service delivery. In Northern California, from San Jose to San Francisco, there are ten places that do cardiovascular surgery outside of Kaiser Permanente. Four of them have significantly lower volume than is recommended. They don't coordinate their efforts, but patients don't know that, and the hospitals are not going to tell them. Health care in this country remains a nineteenth-century cottage industry. It's physicians in small offices and every community hospital for itself.

THE DECLINING ROLE OF GOVERNMENT: IT'S TIME TO PREPARE

PHILIP A. PIZZO, M.D., is dean of the Stanford School of Medicine. Formerly, he was the physician-in-chief of Children's Hospital in Boston and chair of the Department of Pediatrics at Harvard Medical School. He served as chief of the National Cancer Institute's pediatric department, and was acting scientific director for NCI's Division of Clinical Sciences.

RS: **Do you think Medicare will continue to fund graduate medical education?**

PIZZO: All of us in academic medicine ought to be getting ready for that funding to be seriously challenged, probably in the next decade and certainly before 2016 when the Medicare trust fund is going to get into serious trouble. I doubt that policymakers at risk for the wrath of seniors would prioritize GME over direct care. So one way or the other, teaching hospitals are going to have to accommodate for this training. I don't think we are prepared for it. We live in denial.

> *All of us in academic medicine ought to be getting ready for Medicare funding to be seriously challenged, probably in the next decade.*

Unfortunately, this is one of the few profit centers that exist in some states. Hospitals that are struggling to provide some margin would really look askance at giving up that source of funding. That doesn't mean there won't be federal support for GME. The analogy is support that has come to children's hospitals through a different appropriation process.

RS: **Some economists think funding for GME is unnecessary because residents are delivering care to people who are uninsured or who have expensive, complicated illnesses. It's almost like a case-mix adjustment for the payment the hospital gets. Like the old guild model, the difference between what residents could make and what they do make is their implied tuition.**

PIZZO: First of all, after four years of medical school, you're not competent to practice medicine. As I'm teaching residents, I watch their information base grow over time. I could argue that carefully graduated, supervised training is essential to assure quality and safety. But exactly where the money goes, after salaries are paid, is a big black box in many academic centers, quite honestly. And we've never been able to wrestle out the budget for GME from our affiliated teaching hospitals.

RS: So there's a disincentive to make changes.
PIZZO: If there were a 12 percent withdrawal of those funds, just as there was in 1997 with the Balanced Budget Act, I think a lot of teaching hospitals would slip below their margin and get into trouble very quickly. You can't remove $20 to $50 million and expect you're going to find that someplace else.

RS: Would that impact teaching?
PIZZO: You have to realize that most physicians have a significant portion of their compensation at risk. They're expected to generate more clinical productivity and relative value units, so spending time on teaching impacts negatively on their own financial well-being. It's hard to get people to spend time doing it.

RS: Well, suppose we cut down the amount of direct medical education (DME) payments. It totals about $8 to $10 billion, depending on the year and the arithmetic. If we pulled it out, there would have to be a transition.
PIZZO: Right, and that was attempted in New York. It didn't work.

RS: Do you support the AAMC recommendations to substantially increase the supply of doctors?
PIZZO: First, the concept that one is going to solve the problems in certain specialty or geographic or primary care areas, just because you increase the number of people going to medical school, is not supported by decades worth of data. The reality is that graduating physicians choose to go into certain areas on the basis of a whole variety of reasons that may vary considerably from those that they entered medical school with. And it's not at all clear that residency programs are necessarily matched to population needs, either geographically or by specialty.

So I think the premise that increasing the workforce is going to lead to a solution of the distribution issues is probably fallacious. And there has been no effort to develop residency programs that regulate the distribution. I doubt there would be a willingness to do that.

RS: **Why do you think the recommendations were made?**

PIZZO: Part of the AAMC's reason for increasing the workforce is that they're concerned that the number of graduates of allopathic schools could be eclipsed in the next decade or two by graduates from osteopathic schools or offshore schools.

And the health care system is oriented toward producing specialists of one kind or another; the number of primary care physicians is declining. I don't see how we can change that trend. So other economic models that are emerging, the Wal-Mart model and the GE model, are reactions to the lack of a coherent system.

We don't need to train more doctors. More important to me is the need to have a more rational health care system. I realize I'm talking to an economist, but it seems to me that the experiment of making medicine susceptible to market forces has largely failed, and I don't think it's going to get better with just more market pressures.

> *It seems to me that the experiment of making medicine susceptible to market forces has largely failed.*

RS: **You spoke of the need for primary care doctors. What is Stanford's view on this?**

PIZZO: Stanford is a very research-intensive place, and we're primarily interested in training physician-scientists and physician-leaders. It's a small school. We have eighty-six students a year. If we increased our class size, it would be in order to increase the number of people who would be going into research and academic positions.

TOMORROW'S DOCTORS WANT SOMETHING DIFFERENT

EDWARD S. SALSBERG is a senior associate vice president and the director of the Center for Workforce Studies at the Association of American Medical Colleges (AAMC) in Washington, D.C. He is also on the faculty at the George Washington University Medical Center. Prior to joining AAMC, Mr. Salsberg was the executive director of the Center for Health Workforce Studies, which he established in 1996 at the School of Public Health at the University at Albany of the State University of New York (SUNY).

RS: **Who should pay for medical training?**
SALSBERG: I testified to Medicare at MedPac a few weeks ago, and we do think it's an appropriate responsibility for Medicare, since a good deal of the increased demand is going to be driven by the growing elderly population and their use of services. So, therefore, Medicare has an inherent interest in ensuring an adequate supply of appropriately trained doctors.

RS: **Well some economists suggest that Medicare shouldn't pay for any of the training of doctors, providing we make sure that the uninsured have some place to go. The current situation works out pretty well for the hospital. In fact, there was an experiment in New York a few years ago. Medicare said to the hospitals, "We'll give you the money—but stop training residents." There were a few takers, but then after a couple of years almost all of them said, "We changed our mind. We want the residents."**[28]
SALSBERG: Well, there's a prestige factor for the hospital, and there is an overall economic package factor. If you want to be a first-class hospital, you want to have teaching and research and medical suites. If you don't have residents, you can't get those NIH grants that give you higher prestige and help you recruit the best doctors. The residents need to make a reasonable salary.

RS: **It's true that residents don't make much, but my research on rates of return studies suggests that they make it up later.**
SALSBERG: Yes, but it takes years because of high debt. Other professions do it differently. The major New York law firms are taking kids right out of law school and offering them $160,000. At the same time, we have these medi-

cal students who are finishing their fourth year of school and then have three to five more years at maybe $40,000 or $45,000. So we tell them, "Don't worry. When you're thirty-five, you'll start making good money. You'll have $200,000 in debt and you'll pay it off by the time you're fifty, and then you're going to be in great shape."

> We tell residents, "Don't worry. When you're thirty-five, you'll start making good money. You'll have $200,000 in debt and you'll pay it off by the time you're fifty, and then you're going to be in great shape."

RS: That's a really good point. But medicine is still considered a pretty good deal. We've had roughly two applications for every seat over the last ten years. In fact, I'm told it's going to tick up again. Do you think we'll continue to attract the best and brightest?

SALSBERG: Actually applications have been up 4 or 5 percent for each of the last five years. And the MCAT scores are getting higher.

RS: I wrote a paper years ago with Roger Feldman in which we looked at the applications to medical school and the MCAT scores, and calculated the elasticity to the rate of return to number of seats. As the rate of return goes down, the number of applications goes down, and vice versa. And when the rate of return goes down, the average MCAT scores also go down.[29] That means that the people who decide not to apply to medical school are those with higher MCAT scores. Clearly, then, the best and the brightest leave medicine first.

SALSBERG: In any case, the demand for physicians is rising faster than the supply, and it's already too late for us to try and produce all the doctors we would otherwise want for 2020. If we really thought the solution was M.D.s and D.O.s, we should have started ten years ago, and we didn't. So the only way we're going to fill that gap is—as much as I'd like information technology productivity increases—it's probably going to be through nurse practitioners and physician assistants, who are a lot quicker and easier to train than M.D.s.

RS: What has your research shown about the workforce supply?

SALSBERG: We're very interested in the supply-side factors. We did a survey of active and retired physicians over fifty to look at their practice plans and what factors they considered when thinking about retiring. We also wanted to assess whether the newest generation of physicians will be contributing less work effort than their predecessors. So we surveyed physicians under fifty to look at work hours and attitudes toward their ideal practice. From the younger physicians, we heard lots of anecdotes about not wanting to work the hours that physicians did in the past.

RS: **What can you tell me about trends in retirement?**
SALSBERG: A lot of doctors are now nearing retirement as a result of the doubling of medical school capacity in the 1960s and 1970s. We went from fewer than eight thousand graduates to more than sixteen thousand. That big increase is now thirty, thirty-five years out, and those doctors are getting ready to retire. But there was also a relatively steady increase beginning in 1960 and going to about 1980. We did a direct comparison of the actual retirement rates in the cohort compared to what the older models forecast.

RS: **What did that show?**
SALSBERG: More doctors are going to retire sooner than in the models. Our estimate is that retirements are going to grow from about ten thousand a year in the year 2000 to about twenty thousand a year in 2020, driven by just the increasing age of the workforce. Think about twenty thousand doctors retiring each year. If they all work one year longer, that adds twenty thousand to the pool at any one time. If it's two years, it adds forty thousand. So the decision about when they're going to retire, plus or minus two years, will have an enormous impact on how many physicians are out there practicing in 2025.

> *Think about twenty thousand doctors retiring each year. If they all work one year longer, that adds twenty thousand to the pool at any one time.*

RS: **What are some of the factors physicians take into consideration in deciding when to retire?**
SALSBERG: There are external factors that will have a major impact. For some doctors it will be income. If the stock market goes up several thousand points, some will retire. If regulation of medicine gets too heavy they may leave. Or if malpractice liability expense gets too much. My personal sense is

that the nation is going to face a shortage if we don't pay more attention to what older doctors want.

One of the interesting things is the extent to which older doctors want the same things as the younger ones—more flexibility in scheduling, less evenings and weekends, the ability to come in and practice medicine and do less paperwork. Group practices, hospitals, and maybe HMOs can provide far more support services to physicians.

RS: What is the thinking behind the AAMC's recommendation for more medical schools and GME slots?

SALSBERG: We recommended the increase in undergraduate education in large part because we were concerned about physician shortages. While I would love to see less reliance on IMGs, if our long-range goal is to increase the physician supply, it's going to require not only an increase in medical doctors and doctors of osteopathy, but some continuation of IMGs. Even if the AAMC recommendations are followed, this is not going to meet all the demand that we expect to be out there. Of course if we reduced administrative time and paperwork, that could lead to a major increase in physician hours available—without adding one additional doctor.

THE MEDICAL HOME AND OTHER WAYS
TO SAVE PRIMARY CARE

STEVEN SCHROEDER, M.D., is Distinguished Professor of Health and Health Care, Division of General Internal Medicine, Department of Medicine, at the University of California, San Francisco, and also heads the Smoking Cessation Leadership Center. Between 1990 and 2002 he was president and CEO of the Robert Wood Johnson Foundation. He has published extensively in the fields of clinical medicine, health care financing and organization, prevention, public health, and the workforce.

RS: **How do you think managed care changed the functioning of health care delivery?**

SCHROEDER: Managed care made people conscious of ways to save money, and it created business opportunities for people who are managing the care. Most of these opportunities are in the areas of managing, submitting, and verifying claims, not really managing care. So it's not a myth that under managed care physicians spend a lot more time writing their medical records, doing their billing, handling the bill turn-downs, resubmitting claims.

All this created a new function of work in medicine that hardly existed previously. Also, it created a fair bit of irritation because companies have an incentive to pay as little as possible and to hold the money as long as possible. So there's more of a push and pull between the billers and the payers, especially with the higher-volume, lower-dollar per-case clinical practices. If you're only doing five really expensive cases per week, that's different than if you're doing a hundred cheaper ones. That's another reason why the primary care folks are yelping more than, for example, the interventional radiologists.

RS: **Do you agree that it wasn't Halley's Comet that caused the rate of increase of health care spending as a percentage of GNP to slow during the early managed care period?**

SCHROEDER: I think there were two factors for that. First, the economy was booming, so the denominator was growing much faster than it normally does. Second was the constellation of things that we call managed care, which slowed growth in the numerator.

RS: Definitely. But when the economy grows strongly with a lag, health care spending goes up more quickly, not less. So if you have a 2 percent increase in GDP, you may get a 3 or 3.5 percent increase in health care spending.

SCHROEDER: But if the economy had not grown as fast over those seven or eight years, it would have looked like we'd gone from 13 to 15 percent faster. All I know is the GDP is the denominator, and if the denominator is growing faster, all things being equal, the total fraction doesn't go up.

RS: How do you think reimbursement strategies impact the balance between primary care and the specialties?

SCHROEDER: The primary care function is in real peril for a variety of reasons, at least some of them reimbursement-based. Economists don't want to touch it because they say the market determines what happens. But in health care the market is very imperfect because the prices are really set by what's essentially a cartel of medical specialists. It's very heavily weighted toward the procedures. The so-called cognitive specialties like internal medicine, family medicine, and psychiatry each get one vote even though altogether they probably represent half the doctors in the country.

> *The market is very imperfect because the prices are really set by what's essentially a cartel of medical specialists.*

All the intervention specialties like radiotherapists, intervention radiologists, regular radiologists, and all the others get one vote each. So the votes come out something like twenty-five to three in favor of intervention. This is much more true in the U.S. than in other countries. And there is a creep factor so that the updates get captured by the specialist.

RS: Is this like the relative value scale for Medicare?

SCHROEDER: Yes, but it's not just Medicare because all the health insurers take their cue from it. So hourly income for primary care is something like half of what technology-intensive procedures get. And it's gotten worse with increasing medical student debt, the appeal of shift work, and the fear that being in a generalist field spreads you way too thin.

Hospitals see their bottom line as getting quaternary references—that is, beyond tertiary cases. So they make those specialty areas really nice, but for the primary care providers, it's sort of a shabby basement. Then the students who work there see that those are not comparable kinds of experiences, and even the students who really want to do primary care can get turned off.

RS: **What can we do about primary care?**

SCHROEDER: The medical home concept is an attempt to say that we need to build in some incentive structures for the primary care and/or coordinated care function that is so necessary to managing complex chronic illness. And we can value primary care more at the medical schools, in residencies, and in the public. There are lots of pressure points where this can happen. You can do debt relief for students who go into primary care. There are probably ten or fifteen things you could do.

RS: **You're an internist yourself. How does your specialty see these issues?**

SCHROEDER: Actually, Harold Sox and I recently wrote an editorial in the *Annals of Internal Medicine* in which we talked about that. It basically says that internists should either get serious about primary care or get out of it.[30]

RS: **Do you think we should continue to depend heavily on IMGs?**

SCHROEDER: The critical question is that, at the margin, would the U.S. be better off and would those countries be better off if we admitted more U.S. medical students? We graduate about sixteen thousand allopathic physicians, two thousand osteopaths, and we have twenty-five thousand first-year residency positions. So you can do the math. There could be economic incentives, as there were in the 1970s and 1980s, to increase the number of medical students. But I think the current incentives are immoral. Of the industrialized countries, only the U.S. and the U.K. do this to a great extent. It's much less than 15 percent for Sweden, Switzerland, France, and other places.

Would the U.S. be better off and would those countries be better off if we admitted more U.S. medical students?

RS: **Some of the OECD countries keep it down to around 10 percent.**

SCHROEDER: I agree, but you know morality doesn't test by quantity. If you kill a hundred people or you kill one, it's still immoral. It's hard to split immoral.

RS: So what should we do in terms of residencies?

SCHROEDER: I think we need better balance between the number of American graduates and the number of residency positions. We could do that either by increasing the number of graduates—and many are now advocating that—or by reducing the number of residency positions. Or by a combination of both.

RS: I see. So there wouldn't be room for any IMGs?

SCHROEDER: I think they should compete. Let the hospital decide.

RS: That would be a nightmare. It would mean that some of our own graduates would be prevented from entering tax-subsidized residency programs in favor of foreign-trained people. That's a tough policy.

SCHROEDER: Theoretically, that could happen now.

EXTERNAL REPORTING AND OTHER KEYS TO P4P

STEPHEN M. SHORTELL, PH.D., is the Blue Cross of California Distinguished Professor of Health Policy and Management and Professor of Organization Behavior at the School of Public Health and Haas School of Business at the University of California, Berkeley. He is also the dean of the School of Public Health at Berkeley. He is a past editor of *Health Services Research* and has served as president of the Association for Health Services Research.

RS: **What do you think of the use of incentives in medical care?**

SHORTELL: I'm convinced that differential financial incentives to reward providers is a good idea. It's also fraught with danger, because the devil's always in the details, and there are a lot of details when it comes to differentiating performance and paying according to that.

> *The devil's always in the details, and there are a lot of details when it comes to differentiating performance and paying according to that.*

RS: **So what are some of the things we need to know about?**

SHORTELL: Well, one has to do with incentive size—how much does it take to motivate changes in behavior? We don't have a good idea about that. Second, at what level should we place the reward? Should it be at the organizational level and let them do as they wish with the money? Should it be at the group or team level? Or do you go down to the individual doctor level? There are pros and cons involving all of them.

The third question is whether you reward for meeting absolute thresholds of quality metrics that individuals or groups achieve, or also for improvement over time. There could even be hybrid models, whereby you don't get any reward unless you hit a certain threshold. So, for example, with breast cancer screening, everybody should reach about 80 percent of eligible women, so you don't get anything unless you hit that, even if the year before you were at 40 percent and improved to 60 percent. In contrast there might be other metrics in which you hit a threshold, say it's 50 percent, and then above that an additional reward for improvement kicks in.

So there needs to be experimentation around the various models.

RS: Uwe Reinhardt says the levels of incentives so far are just too small.

SHORTELL: I agree. It's also possible that external reporting has a bigger impact. There was a very nice randomized study in Wisconsin involving three groups of hospitals. One group got no feedback at all. A second group got feedback, but it was kept inside the hospital. The third group's performance was publicly reported. The most improvement was in the latter group. It was a step function.

RS: So is that where you think pay for performance ought to go?

SHORTELL: Yes, I think it has to be combined with external reporting and a portfolio of incentives, not just money.

RS: In addition to bonuses, some places are giving grants to see if that works. And some people prefer the stick to the carrot, saying you should just penalize providers if they don't make the benchmarks. What do you think of that?

SHORTELL: I don't know whether there's a lot of evidence for this, but my sense is that with professionals like doctors, penalties or withholds don't go down well. It's better to go with positive rewards. The formula for Medicare is designed to be budget neutral; so if they employ some kind of P4P in the doctor sector, there will have to be winners and losers. One thing that's being talked about is reallocating the money and putting some percentage of it into a quality improvement competitive pool.

RS: That would be a withhold.

SHORTELL: Yes, and you can view it as a penalty I suppose, but everybody is at the starting gate. They are all eligible to get that money. So it will go to the higher performers.

RS: In addition to Medicare, I understand that a lot of the Medicaid programs are also gearing up for P4P. So it's happening not only at the national level, but at the state level. You were very involved in the one in California. Tell me about that.

SHORTELL: California's was one of the earlier programs and is the largest. It's unusual because we got all—and I mean *all*—of the major insurers around the table with the lead medical groups, and with some consumer reps, to agree to a standardized set of measures and reporting. And that wasn't easy.

RS: All that must have taken some finesse.

SHORTELL: It took a lot of discussion and willingness to compromise among those involved. We had to move gingerly because different health plans have their own wrinkle on the bonus and how it's constructed. But importantly, they all agreed on a single reporting and data-collection configuration, using the same numerator and denominator. There is some evidence of steady, if not large, progress on most of the quality indicators over time. The groups are now exploring the use of efficiency and care coordination measures as well.

WHAT THE BUSINESS MODEL
AND THE MILITARY MODEL KNOW

MARK D. SMITH, M.D., is president and CEO of the California HealthCare Foundation. He is a member of the clinical faculty at the University of California, San Francisco, and an attending physician at the Positive Health Program for AIDS care at San Francisco General Hospital. He has served on the Performance Measurement Committee of the National Committee for Quality Assurance.

RS: Do you agree that when physician income declines in a specialty, it is indicating an oversupply?

SMITH: I think that's probably true over the long term. You can look at the rise and fall of radiology, for instance. But there are two other mechanisms that need to be considered. First, because their incomes are dependent on their control over the practice model, physicians' incomes can be threatened by substitution. There's no better example of that than anesthesiology. What used to be done by anesthesiologists is now done by nurse anesthetists. So the anesthesiologist's income is vulnerable not only to a supply-and-demand mechanism, but also to substitution.

> The anesthesiologist's income is vulnerable not only to a supply-and demand-mechanism, but also to substitution.

RS: What about control over newer technologies?

SMITH: This is important for specialists who have very high incomes. For instance, to the extent that gastroenterologists' income is dependent on doing colonoscopies, the threat from virtual colonoscopy by MRI or other means is significant. So the rise and fall of certain specialties or subspecialties might be based on their ability to make money doing, say, cardiac arrhythmia ablations, or other micro-niches that depend on new technologies. That's why turf wars can be so hard fought. So it's not just supply and demand in terms of numbers. I think it's also how well-protected physicians are against substitution and the extent to which they can get excess "rents" (as you economists would call it), because of their control over certain new technology.

RS: **That's beautifully said, and I think it's exactly right. Do you think P4P will make a difference?**

SMITH: I think it's an excellent idea, and the Foundation has been involved a lot. But it's still early days, and it's still a fairly weak signal. If 5 percent of your income is attributable to P4P and 95 percent is attributable to pay for volume, we shouldn't be surprised if the results are not dramatic. Second, I think the scope of medical practice that is currently under the P4P umbrella is still relatively small and is not, frankly, in place in the parts of medicine that cost a lot of money.

We can do P4P for primary care docs' management of diabetes—whose costs have not increased dramatically from one year to another. But we don't have P4P for cardiac ablation, joint replacement, spinal devices, or any of the places where you've seen explosions in costs, in part related to indication creep and volume creep. It's like looking under the street lamp for the keys because that's where the light is. We do P4P where we have good measurement, but we don't have good measurement in the places where much of the financial action is.

We do P4P where we have good measurement, but we don't have good measurement in the places where much of the financial action is.

RS: **Since P4P is pretty much paid at the medical group level, the incentives trickling down to the doctor don't have much impact.**

SMITH: Well, part of what happened with capitation is that it withered on the vine. Various parties agreed to get a lot of the areas with the most dramatic increases carved out of the capitation rate. The best example of that is joint replacement surgery, where the increases are mainly going to the device companies. The total payment has risen dramatically over the last fifteen years, but the portion that goes to the hospital has stayed about constant. The portion that goes to the doctor has decreased. The portion that has increased has *not* gone to the insurance company; it's gone to the medical device firm. That's true in all of these areas, whether it's cardiac stents or spinal devices.

RS: **I know you've spent some time looking at the efficiency of health care in the military. What can we learn from that?**

SMITH: In an environment with a life-and-death imperative, and in the absence of litigation, people can do a lot more than they're allowed to do in most of civilian life. There are ways to get around problems, particularly the shortages that result from lack of physical presence in a given location. So as you might expect, the most advanced telemetry medicine in the world is practiced in the military.

They've got suits that can remotely monitor the vital signs of someone who's been injured. And on submarines that don't surface for months at a time, they have 150 sailors who are taken care of by someone who's got six months to a year of training, plus backup by telephone.

RS: So is this a model that can make its way to the nonmilitary sector, just like the medics did with physician assistants?
SMITH: Well, as we know, physician assistants have hardly revolutionized health care. It's more of a niche development that's marginally been assimilated, as opposed to fundamentally changing the model. The pressure to reduce cost has not been sufficient to overcome the conservatism of the system and the hegemony of the guilds. Systems like Kaiser can internalize these trade-offs, and have, for example, well-trained nurses doing colonoscopies rather than gastroenterologists.

RS: Why do you think so many innovations originate in the military?
SMITH: There's a kind of semipermeable membrane between the military system and the civilian system. Throughout civilian care there are dozens of innovations that could have diffused and lowered costs but did not. The problem is not finding innovations; the problem is that there are so many interests that stifle innovation if it's not accompanied by indemnification of the incumbents. It's what I call Health Care Whack-A-Mole.

RS: Okay. How does Health Care Whack-A-Mole work?
SMITH: Lots of examples. Retail clinics pop up, and the AMA tries to whack them down. Specialty hospitals pop up, and the general hospitals try to stamp them out. The argument is always, "We

Retail clinics pop up, and the AMA tries to whack them down. Specialty hospitals pop up, and the general hospitals try to stamp them out.

shouldn't allow innovation unless you can guarantee that I will not be hurt." There is no other industry in which that's the statement going in.

RS: So inefficiency and costs stay in the system. Some people say we could get 50 percent more productivity out of it. But others caution that medicine is not like engineering or manufacturing. It's a personal service that requires a trusting relationship between the patient and doctor.

SMITH: I think that is largely wishful thinking. A lot of medicine is quite similar to engineering and manufacturing. They are more or less industrial processes. Are there parts of medicine where there's a close personal relationship involved? Of course. But not always: Have you had a colonoscopy in the last ten years?

RS: Oh, I had one.

SMITH: Did you have a close personal relationship with the gastroenterologist?

RS: No.

SMITH: Right. Most people don't see the need for a close personal relationship with the optometrist who checks the pressure in their eye, but do want one with their psychiatrist or their child's pediatrician. There are clearly areas that are as reducible to time, motion, and efficiency as any other service. And there are parts that are truly unique. What we need is a system that recognizes which is which, and deploys people, including physicians, where their training and expense are appropriate.

RS: What do you see in terms of substitution in the future?

There are a lot of personal services that we now do for ourselves that at one time required highly paid intermediaries with specialized technical knowledge.

SMITH: There are a lot of personal services that we now do for ourselves that at one time required highly paid intermediaries with specialized technical knowledge. We don't even think twice about making an airline reservation or buying a stock. The question for the future is the extent to which we will remove the intermediaries in health care in the same way we've removed them in other personal service industries. Of course there are safety concerns that need to be taken very seriously. On the other hand, I'll bet there isn't a single stock broker or travel agent who wouldn't have said twenty years ago, "You can't let people trade their own stocks; they'll all go broke in a minute. They need the protection of my system, my license, and my expertise in order for the world to stay on its axis."

RS: **Do you think we have too few or too many doctors?**

SMITH: It's hard to know how many doctors we need, because we underappreciate the pace of scientific change and we overappreciate the capacity of the profession to protect its own income and avoid replacement by lower-cost devices or people. I was struck by an article that Ezekiel Emanuel wrote about the nature of premedical requirements.[31] He points out that for a young person to become a doctor, he or she has to take, and excel in, physics and organic chemistry, but not psychology or organizational development. These requirements are really rooted in the notion of doctor as independent scientist-investigator, which is not actually what most doctors are.

RS: **Right, you have to study calculus to be a doctor.**

SMITH: And I can teach you the calculus you need to know to be a doctor in the twenty-first century in about two weeks. The whole notion of creating physician scientists is rooted in a failure to understand the role of the modern doctor. This is especially true in the field of primary care, which is really struggling for an identity and for a viable future. But if you ask most of the primary care true advocates what it is that those docs will be doing in the future, the response is usually "managing complex chronic disease" and "guiding patient behavior." But I'm doubtful that we can produce a physician workforce that's competent at these tasks, having selected them for their competence in calculus and physics.

> *The whole notion of creating physician scientists is rooted in a failure to understand the role of the modern doctor.*

MORE DOCTORS DOES NOT EQUAL BETTER OUTCOMES

JOHN E. WENNBERG, M.D., is the Peggy Y. Thomson Chair in the Evaluative Clinical Sciences and director emeritus of the Dartmouth Institute for Health Policy and Clinical Practice. He is a professor in Dartmouth's Department of Community and Family Medicine and in the Department of Medicine. He is the founding editor of *The Dartmouth Atlas of Health Care*, which examines medical resource intensity and utilization in the United States.

RS: You've done pioneering work in evaluating medical practice. Do you think pay for performance will work well?

WENNBERG: One of our critiques of P4P is that it is focused on the underuse of effective care. In other words, did you do your beta blockers? In these cases, patient preference isn't a factor. But this is a really small proportion of medical care for the Medicare population—about 12 percent of spending if you just count people being hospitalized for certain cancer surgical procedures, heart attacks, strokes, broken hips—things for which a certain treatment almost always makes sense.

RS: How should the focus of pay for performance be expanded?

WENNBERG: It needs to deal with the overuse and misuse of care. About 60 percent of Medicare spending is associated with the capacity of the system; we call those supply-sensitive services. An example would be the frequency with which you have the chronic illness patient revisit the physician. With congestive heart failure, you might see the patient every six weeks or every twelve weeks. There are no rules and no evidence that governs frequency of revisit. So capacity dominates. If you have more cardiologists, the effect of the population at risk is to cut the interval between revisits by about half.

> We believe that four out of five knee replacement operations are on the wrong patient—on patients who don't want the operation.

Another 25 or 30 percent is for what we call preference-sensitive care: for example, procedures like knee replacements or hip replacements, where patient preferences play a big role—or should—in determining the medical necessity. As things now stand, we believe that four out of five knee replacement operations are on the wrong patient—on patients who don't want the operation.

RS: Okay, would you repeat that for me?

WENNBERG: You heard it right. This estimate is based on a very nice population-based, Canadian study that used appropriateness criteria to estimate the need for surgery.[32] Surgical need was defined clinically as patients with significant pain and X-ray evidence for a deformity that indicates that the patient could benefit from replacement. If those things exist, the patient would be eligible for surgery according to the clinical appropriateness criteria.

But then the researchers introduced the additional requirement that medical necessity be defined by the patient's own preference for treatment. It turned out that only 15 percent of the patients in that study actually wanted surgery. They much preferred to live with their problem for the time being. So "demand" for surgery based on clinical criteria exceeded by a factor of four or five the amount that informed patients wanted. The implication is that if you just use the appropriateness factor, you'll be operating on patients who don't want the procedure four times out of five.

What pay for performance should pay for is decisions that ensure that the patients who want to get operated on are the ones who do get operated on. CMS should require that certified decision aids be used to inform patients about treatment choices.

RS: You are well known for your work on decision aids. Can you say a bit about them?

WENNBERG: Over the years we've designed a series of decision aids—they're mostly videos now—that basically tell patients about their treatment options, what's known and not known about the risks and benefits, and why it's important that patients get involved. More than fifty clinical trials have been completed showing that patients who use decision aids make high-quality decisions. There's an industry around them now, updating these tools and making sure they're authentic. Most times, when patients are more aware of their options, the rates of procedures go down, which is potentially good for the health care economy.

Most times, when patients are more aware of their options, the rates of procedures go down, which is potentially good for the health care economy.

RS: **Tell me how you measure the quality.**

WENNBERG: Questionnaires reveal whether or not patients were informed and whether the choices they made reflected their underlying values and concerns. Breast cancer is a good example. Decision quality measures reveal whether the patient knew that women who have a lumpectomy face the possibility that the cancer will come back locally and most need radiation. Some women don't want to have to undergo surveillance for recurrence and they may not want to have radiation, so therefore they may prefer a mastectomy. Other women just really don't want to lose their breast and so they'll take those risks for recurrence and radiation. Relating these concerns to the decisions actually made is integral to measuring decision quality.

RS: **How would pay for performance move into the chronic care model?**

WENNBERG: Well, that's a different sort of story. Here the problem is unwarranted variation in supply-sensitive care and the fact that capacity is deployed very differently across markets. For example, Los Angeles has lots of beds and doctors, and its physicians put many people in the hospital and provide many more visits and diagnostic tests than do providers in Sacramento. My colleagues and I have recently proposed that CMS encourage reduction in overuse of care by rewarding providers who effectively coordinate care and reduce excess hospitalizations.[33]

The emphasis on science is important. If you ask what the best protocols are for managing congestive heart failure—whether Los Angeles is closer to it than Sacramento, for example—the scientific community provides no answer. But the emphasis on reducing overuse comes from epidemiologic studies that suggest the more frequent use of supply-sensitive care isn't better. This comes from the work of Elliott Fisher and colleagues.[34] They looked at cohorts of patients with conditions that require hospitalization and that can be treated—things like hip fractures, acute myocardial infarction, and operable colon cancers—and followed those patients for up to five years afterward. They found a consistently higher mortality rate among people who live in regions with high rates of use of care, such as Los Angeles, compared to people who live in low-use regions, such as Sacramento. There is about a 5 percent higher mortality rate associated with one's use of care.

RS: What is the thinking on the reasons for this difference?

WENNBERG: Well, for one thing, if you hospital-ize people twice as often, they have twice as many chances of medical error.

If you hospitalize people twice as often, they have twice as many chances of medical error.

RS: What does your work on variation say about the need to increase the physician workforce?

WENNBERG: I certainly don't recommend an increase in the physician supply until we know a good deal more about what works and what patients want.

Given the current disequilibrium between supply and utilization, the number of physicians who can find gainful employment—and practice to accepted clinical guidelines or practice styles—seems to exceed the number available in all parts of the United States.

The problem can be traced to the way we pay for care. We have a health care system that pays for utilization. In many parts of the country, the workforce is unchecked by any kind of planning. Now, Kaiser has a reason-ably strict way of deciding how many doctors it needs, and it's based on the population it serves. There's not much variation between the Kaiser plans in terms of the numbers of doctors employed and their mix between special-ties. However, if you look at most of the systems in the country, you see huge differences in the quantities and the types of physicians that are employed to manage chronic illness, and also differences between regions and age differ-ences of surgeons. So if you're talking about a needs-based model of planning for physician capacity, you get stuck at first base. You should use benchmarks, at least to understand what the variation is in the way the workforce is de-ployed. The Dartmouth Atlas is full of benchmarks.[35]

If you want to use current practice to predict how many doctors you need, you soon find out that if you use cities like New York or Miami as a standard, you would have to increase the number of doctors by 34 to 40 percent to bring the rest of the country up to that standard, just to meet today's "need" for physicians. But if you take the Mayo Clinic and their use of workforce as your standard, you have more than enough to meet today's need as well as the expected increase in the number of older Americans as the baby boomer generation enters Medicare.

DOCTORS AS TEAM PLAYERS

WILLIAM J. BARCELLONA is vice president for government affairs at the California Association of Physician Groups. He serves as adjunct professor with the University of Southern California's School of Policy, Planning, and Development, teaching management of health care organizations. Formerly, he was deputy director of California's Department of Managed Health Care, where he drafted health care legislation, including the continuity of care law (SB244).

RS: **Tell me about California's physician groups and how they developed.**
BARCELLONA: There was a tremendous shake-out among risk-bearing physician groups from about 1998 to 2002. Something like 110 of them either closed or merged into other groups. And consequent to the financial solvency regulations, all the risk-bearing organizations now report financial status. It's been a lot more stable since then. There's maybe one closure a year out of about 300 active groups in the state. Since capitation rates have stabilized, that's allowed these groups to coalesce and prosper. About 75 percent of all HMO membership is in the largest 30 or so groups.

RS: **What's been the effect on primary care providers in groups?**
BARCELLONA: In the full IPA model, where the entire network is contracted around an administrative core, the doctors at the PCP level are hardest hit.

In the medical group model, we're seeing bumped-up salaries to bring in younger doctors, particularly in the tougher urban areas.

In the medical group model, where they're employed, we're seeing bumped-up salaries to bring in younger doctors, particularly in the tougher urban areas. It's particularly tricky to track specialists because one person may be contracted in five or six different networks.

We recently prepared a report that shows all of our member groups, and the split between PCPs versus specialists in each group. It adds up to about twenty thousand PCPs in the 150 member groups.

RS: **How is pay for performance working in California?**
BARCELLONA: It's focused on primary care. I think we're some distance away from really rolling that out into the specialist networks. Some of the

groups are all primary care doctors, and then they contract with the specialty networks. Then you've got Hill Physicians, which has an entire contracted network of PCPs and specialists, and so there's another way for them to distribute it.

RS: **How do they get the productivity out of the group? Productivity to an economist means less input for the same amount of output.**
BARCELLONA: Increased productivity means removing the administrative barriers so the doctors can see more patients, but it also means making the visits more efficient. It could mean telemedicine. It could mean communicating with your patients through email, adopting EMR technology, that sort of thing. So there are really several different levels.

RS: **How do the groups feel about the idea of a shorter visit?**
BARCELLONA: That bothers them. On the other hand, eliminating unnecessary visits can be very, very beneficial. You can handle some things in an email or pass it on to an NP. What I hear from our members is a lot of enthusiasm around getting more mid-level practitioners into the mix. They believe there's a shortage of doctors in California, and they think this will help.

DOCTORS: STOP BEING DEPRESSED
AND REDESIGN THE SYSTEM

IAN MORRISON, PH.D., is president emeritus of the Institute for the Future and chair of its Health Advisory Panel. He is a past director of the Health Research and Education Trust (HRET) of the American Hospital Association. He is a director of the Center for Health Design and of the California HealthCare Foundation. He also serves as a member of the Stakeholders Advisory Committee of the Program for Health Systems Improvement at Harvard University.

RS: From your vantage point as a health care futurist, how do you think managed care and its aftermath have worked out for doctors?

MORRISON: My experience working with physicians is they're all clinically depressed. They feel like hamsters on a treadmill, and they're going faster and faster trying to get to their target income. I wrote a piece with Richard Smith for the *British Medical Journal* years ago called "Hamster Health Care."[36] I think it's true that in the developed countries, discounted fee for service has made doctors feel like hamsters on a treadmill. And it's a profound and annoying irony for doctors when they see all these hangers-on such as futurists like me and random health CEOs and salesmen for pharmaceutical companies making way more money than they are.

I think there's been an astonishing lack of leadership by the physician community in engaging in the transformation of health care delivery.

I have sympathy for their frustration, but I also think there's been an astonishing lack of leadership by the physician community in engaging in the transformation of health care delivery.

With the exception of the doctors who have drunk the Kool-Aid—Don Berwick and Jack Wennberg and Elliott Fisher and others—I would estimate that only 5 to 10 percent of all physicians believe transformation is necessary and possible. There's a significant majority who wish it were 1975 again.

RS: Well, it wasn't long after 1975 that the so-called managed care revolution got established. That's when doctors were given a set of rules to play by.

MORRISON: Right. And I think it's important to emphasize that the model we've come to today is a perfect hamster care model. More selective contracting. Every doctor is in every network, and the HMOs and health plans have all consolidated to the point that they just beat them up on price. It's in marked contrast to what's happened to the incomes of other professionals in American life.

RS: You talk to physician groups a lot. What do they tell you about managed care and their reaction to it?
MORRISON: Well, it's been a long time since the first big wave hit the East Coast. At the time a lot of us had a positive vision of managed care as capitation and group practice formation. The problem was that, east of the Rockies—with the exception of Geisinger and Mayo and a few isolated examples—there really wasn't a tradition of group practice. This was particularly true in the South. A lot of doctors hated the concept of capitation, or being in groups, or being excluded by a tight PPO. It was doctors who led the charge, through their patients, to create the managed care backlash. And this led to open networks. Ironically, it was this that resulted in more rapidly declining incomes. If you're going to have everybody in, you've got to grind down on price, and that's what happened.

I've come to believe that the selection and training of physicians is really about trying to help smart people make decisions in the middle of the night all by themselves. It's true that many doctors hang on to that sort of image of themselves. They do not do "group" real well. They don't think in process terms much, and they really would like to be left alone and not have people telling them what to do.

> *I've come to believe that the selection and training of physicians is really about trying to help smart people make decisions in the middle of the night all by themselves.*

But I don't think their model is sustainable. I keep talking and writing about the need for reengineering. Doctors come up to me and say, "Who the hell are you—a geography undergraduate—to tell me what to do?" My response is, "You're absolutely right. I just wish you folks would do it. I don't see many of you with good ideas or interest in reengineering the system so that it's faster, better, and cheaper."

RS: **What if they don't?**

MORRISON: My worst nightmare is that their legitimate fear of sustained erosion in their incomes, fear of government, fear of large players, and fear of their own inadequacies as managers will result in the AMA and others resisting any kind of measurement or improvement. And simultaneously they may be unwilling to expand residency programs much because they're worried about short-term competition. In that case we would get the worst of all possible worlds—not enough specialists, and a huge lack of service for lower-income people. I worry about that scenario happening. Not as a planned future, but as a default because people are trying to optimize their behavior for the short run.

RS: **What will happen with measurement of performance?**

MORRISON: I think we're going to have more of it. And there will be transparency. What's going to happen is one of two things. Either the specialty societies are going to step up and put in place peer-to-peer measurement and reporting and feedback systems, or Google is going to do it to them and they're not going to like it.

Either the specialty societies are going to step up and put in place measurement and reporting systems, or Google is going to do it to them and they're not going to like it.

RS: **What can you add to the various forecasts of the supply of doctors?**

MORRISON: I think we should be making aspirational forecasts—setting goals. We want a delivery system with the following characteristics. It's almost reverse engineering. We should be encouraging different skill sets to emerge, and to be much more innovative in the way we do care and delivery. Otherwise, the one thing that's for sure is that it's going to cost a lot more.

RS: **What are the skill sets you think we need?**

MORRISON: What we really need is the sort of physician leader who can manage other physicians. I'm swayed by the Mayo Clinics and the Kaisers and the Virginia Masons of the world and a lot of hospital systems that are run by really smart physicians who know that they have to get their physician colleagues with the program. We need to move from 1 percent of all physicians as leaders to 50 percent who have an aptitude, interest, and some ability in that area.

RS: **Until we do that, what do you see in terms of shortages and surpluses of doctors?**

MORRISON: I see that it's becoming increasingly difficult to get specialists because we blew off gatekeepers. Everywhere I go they can't get them, particularly in high-cost areas. Kaiser has no trouble getting folks because they're paying people a reasonably high salary and there's no heavy lifting. No on-call, no weekends, it's manageable. So you can have a life. But at a place like the Palo Alto Medical Clinic, it's hard to get specialists to move there because of high home prices and all the rest of it. And even though we've moved away from the gatekeeper model, we're seeing a collapse of primary care. At a hospital retreat that I conducted, they told me that the average age of primary care doctors in their network is sixty-three.

RS: **Do you see a solution?**

MORRISON: Actually, I think we need to redesign care delivery in a very profound way, including using much less expensive alternatives. And specialists should not be threatened by it because, even if we wanted to, we couldn't train enough specialists between now and when the baby boom hits a wall.

We're missing a huge opportunity for productivity improvement where we could build multidisciplinary teams. If doctors want to lead them, and if they can demonstrate they've got the skills to lead teams, fine. But in a time of scarcity we should not be protecting procedures that could be delegated to other people.

But there are big societal questions about whether we should just overlay the current delivery system and pump up the numbers based on demographic and utilization forecasts. In my opinion, that would lead to a real problem.

RS: **What is the biggest problem from patients' point of view?**

MORRISON: There's an affordability crisis that is large and looming, and we're really struggling with how to address that in a way that's consistent with American values. I think we're in for another round of health reform, and there will be a push for giving people a card for access to a system that is unaffordable. Making people pay $15 grand a year on a health care policy doesn't seem very sensible to me.

RS: Why is the system unaffordable?

> *The phrase I've often used to describe our health care system is the Gong Show.*

MORRISON: The phrase I've often used to describe our health care system is the Gong Show. If you came from another planet and looked at it, you'd say, "Whoever designed this was out of their mind." I'm obviously overstating to make a point. And I am encouraged by the growing recognition about transparency and measurement and trying to align reimbursement systems to performance.

RS: Right. We're open to new things.

MORRISON: Yes, and that's a good thing. The problem is we don't like the smell of the new ideas after a couple of years, and we move on to something else. We're always enamored with the next fad.

A FINAL WORD

At the end of the day, what can we glean from the research set out in Part I of this book and from these extraordinary and insightful conversations with leading figures in the field?

First, from the data analysis in this book and review of recent literature, we know that market indicators—including physician income, selection of specialty, geographic distribution of doctors, and numbers of nonphysician clinicians in the workforce—all respond rapidly and predictably to economic incentives in the marketplace. Further, we know that this is more demonstrably true in the years following the managed care revolution than it was beforehand. Despite the managed care backlash and decline of the past few years, the effect of incentives on physicians, payers, and patients remains potent. Mark Pauly reinforced this view in his comments to me.

Using this knowledge to estimate the "right" supply is nevertheless difficult. As we have seen, forecasting efforts in the past have missed the mark and even led to strategies that caused problems over the long term. Therefore, as a health economist, my inclination is to summarize the input on all sides and leave it at that. (There is some truth in the aphorism that if you laid all the economists end-to-end, they would still not reach a conclusion.)

However, the matter of access to high-quality, cost-effective health care is a crucial challenge to the nation, and determining the size of tomorrow's physician workforce is a key factor, especially given the very high cost of training. Because of the multiyear lag in producing a single new doctor, it is not advisible to wait for certainty that a forecast is exactly right. By then it will be too late to correct a sizable undersupply or oversupply. So decisions must be made under conditions of some uncertainty, and I would like to contribute to that process with the following observations based on the data in this book and generously leavened with the opinions of industry leaders expressed in the Part II conversations.

The overall goal I see is to significantly reduce the imbalance between America's health system costs and the health outcomes it produces. This is what I mean when I refer to the "right" supply of doctors. As we have seen, there is some evidence that having more doctors may not, in fact, get us better health, despite the substantial cost for training and services. Furthermore, John Wennberg's research suggests that a large proportion of medical procedures routinely undertaken by doctors should not be performed—and would *not* be if patients were systematically provided with the information needed to make the best decisions for themselves. Certainly, there is substantial literature in the Dartmouth Atlas[1] and elsewhere purporting to show that regions with more physicians have greater costs but no improvements in patient satisfaction or health outcomes.

By a number of measures, the United States does not stack up well in comparison to other developed nations in either population health or cost-efficiency. The World Health Organization (WHO) published rankings of 191 nations' health systems in 2000.[2] Five performance indicators were used to determine the rankings (not without controversy from some quarters): population health; health inequalities or disparities; health system responsiveness (a combination of patient satisfaction and how well the system acts); distribution of responsiveness across the population; and distribution of the system's financial burden across the population.

France took the highest honors, followed among major countries by Italy, Spain, Austria, and Japan. The United Kingdom was at number 18, Germany at number 25, Canada at number 30, and Australia at number 32. The United States was far down the list in 37th place. This is a notably poor showing, considering the fact that Americans pay a higher percentage of GDP—16 percent—for health care than any other nation. According to the Centers for Medicare & Medicaid Services, health care spending will be over 19 percent of GDP by 2015. As a nation we spend about $8,000 per person for health expenditures, and this is expected to grow to over $12,000 per person by 2015 (in 2007 dollars). During the same period, the money spent on physician and clinical services will rise from about $500 billion in 2008 to some $775 billion in 2015.[3] In his new book *Health Care Reform Now!* George Halvorson notes that five chronic diseases (asthma, congestive heart failure, coronary artery disease, depression, and diabetes) are already responsible for the overwhelming majority of health spending in the U.S.[4]

Mortality and life-expectancy indicators for Americans are also out of step when compared internationally. Johns Hopkins Professor Barbara Starfield compared thirteen countries on sixteen health indicators. The countries were Australia, Belgium, Canada, Denmark, Finland, France, Germany, Japan, the Netherlands, Spain, Sweden, the United Kingdom, and the United States. The average ranking for the United States was 12th—second to last place. On some indicators it came in at the bottom of the list. One of these last-place showings was for neonatal mortality and infant mortality overall.[5]

There are many contributing factors to this poor showing, of course. An important one, according to Starfield and a number of the experts who discussed this with me, is the U.S. overreliance on specialists. Whereas most industrialized countries have roughly half of their physicians in primary care, about two-thirds of the U.S. physician workforce are in specialties.[6] We also know from Starfield's research that regions with more primary care doctors have better health, even after accounting for age and income differences. These regions also have far lower health care costs.[7] The inescapable conclusion is that primary care is better for our overall health and better for our pocketbooks as well. Kevin Grumbach and Jordan Cohen spoke compellingly on this issue.

Unfortunately, primary care in this country does not compare favorably to that in several developed countries, according to a 2006 survey by the Commonwealth Fund. The survey of primary care physicians in Australia, Canada, Germany, New Zealand, the Netherlands, the United Kingdom, and the United States showed that "U.S. physicians are among the least likely to have extensive clinical information systems or incentives targeted on quality, and the most likely to report that their patients have difficulty paying for care."[8] The findings stressed that policy changes could result in better performance.

But nothing happens easily in a health care delivery system riven by competing interests. Those who attempt to influence the supply or role of physicians can find themselves unwilling participants in a game of "Health Care Whack-A-Mole," as Mark Smith of the California HealthCare Foundation puts it. His description of the delivery system is only slightly more upbeat than health futurist Ian Morrison's depiction of "The Gong Show." In fact virtually all of the people I spoke with for this book see systemic complications to ensuring an adequate supply of the right categories of doctors in the right locations over time.

For all of these reasons, *I believe it is productive to frame the doctor supply conversation in a broader, workforce context.* There are more than twelve million health services workers today. Interestingly enough, this is four million more than there were just fifteen years ago. This number doesn't even include the legions of behind-the-scenes health industry workers such as administrative, culinary, technical, and janitorial personnel. By health services workers, I am referring to those on the front lines of care. Health futurist Jeff Goldsmith likes to call them the people who "get blood on their shoes." A relatively small proportion of these are physicians, and in the United States, fewer than half of them are in primary care.

Rather than simply ordering up more doctors, we need integrated solutions that weigh the training and deployment of the entire health services workforce. Aside from the medical procedures that must be performed by a particular type of specialist, health care services can be provided by various combinations of primary care doctors, specialists, nonphysician clinicians, and support personnel. And, very important, much of that work can be performed or greatly facilitated by the use of technology. Arnold Milstein made this point very clearly. The way health care organizations and agencies choose to assemble these players and pay for them to produce a given service determines the price tag. As a nation, we have less and less room for services that cost more than they need to. Our peculiar system wastes a good deal of our resources. If the strain on public programs such as Medicare is not showing now, just wait a few short years until the bulk of the baby boomers reach sixty-five.

With all this in mind, what should America's physician supply look like for the next decade? First, to the extent that we err, it should be on the side of too many doctors as opposed to too few. It is appropriate to allow for a bit of slack because I believe the consequences of having a slight shortage of doctors are worse for the nation's health than having a slight surplus. Further, we need to be prepared for at least some of the state and federal proposals for ramping up health insurance coverage to come to fruition. I would like to see a modest increase of 10 to 20 percent in the production of physicians over the next five to ten years. Both undergraduate slots and residency positions, particularly for primary care doctors, should be increased. To accommodate the lag there may be a need to bring in more international medical graduates.

From an economist's perspective, more important than increasing the numbers of doctors is improving the productivity of those already in place. The health care industry must ensure that doctors produce more high-quality services by putting in place financial and other rewards for doing so. Health care markets, as we have seen, do not easily recognize quality, so it is necessary to have structures in place to do that. Pay for performance, although still in its infancy, can be a powerful tool to ensure that the right things happen to the right patients. P4P can be structured to promote both quality and cost-efficiency, as it is becoming increasingly apparent that the two go hand in hand. In particular, it can strengthen preventive care and patient education. When P4P is paired with transparent measurement and reporting of results, as suggested by Richard Frank, Steve Shortell, and Gail Wilensky, it can strongly influence the decision making of patients as well as doctors. Uwe Reinhardt suggested it's "a two-by-four by which you get the attention of hospital boards."

Pay for performance can also be used to further the medical home, in which patients' primary care setting serves as the hub for coordination of their care and maintains all information relative to their care. The medical home also promotes active collaboration among clinicians. Such collaboration tends to be rewarding for the clinicians, and it is certainly good for patients and families. As my friend and colleague Alain Enthoven puts it: medicine is a team sport. The medical home can and should become more widely supported by payers of all types as the nation's chronic illness rates increase in the near future. To a great extent, the medical home is enabled by comprehensive patient data and communication systems. As other developed nations have demonstrated, such technologies are vital to supporting quality and cost-effectiveness.

Besides pay-for-performance arrangements, health care organizations and policymakers need to encourage innovative ways to pay for health services. Various bundling configurations—the use of a single payment for a group of related services—are being experimented with. This can be thought of as an a la carte menu versus a fixed price one. A bundled payment for inpatient and outpatient care by type of treatment is one mechanism. A further extension of this would be a payment that includes prevention services and health education, which would foster the integration of the workforce.

Because it is clear to me that larger integrated delivery systems are best positioned to offer coordinated, high-quality, cost-effective care, I believe in encouraging the development of these systems and perhaps competition between them. In fact, throughout this book, I have made note of the efficiencies and innovations that have blossomed in such integrated systems. Kaiser Permanente demonstrates one model, but there are others just as viable. Their advances in electronic medical records and networking are perhaps the most compelling. Robert Pearl was passionate about the importance of integration.

My own research and my conversations with various experts convince me that large integrated enterprises are best suited to address a future that will include the retirement years of the baby boomers. The United States will experience a massive demand for chronic care and other services. Unlike previous generations of retirees, this cohort will demand excellent, coordinated, cost-effective, and humane care. As I discussed with Ed Salsberg, this uptick in demand will coincide with an accelerated retirement of doctors—many of whom are themselves boomers. Further diminishing the availability of physicians is the rapidly growing presence of women in medicine. Female physicians tend to work fewer hours on average than males, and are in fact changing workplace norms for the whole profession. More physicians of both sexes are demanding quality-of-life accommodations such as piecework, free weekends, and fewer on-call requirements.

Although all of these factors will significantly change health care delivery, I don't see them as negative. Well-devised policy and payer solutions can lead to a better system overall by paying doctors for what they do best and making greater use of nonphysician health workers, technology, teamwork, and informed self-care. Not only will we pay less for health services, we will be healthier for it.

In the opening chapter of this book, I described an experiment to find correlations between the San Francisco Bay Area's "best" restaurants and "best" doctors. The indicator I used was waiting times for a reservation or an appointment. I found that the "best" doctors, very much like the "best" restaurants, had the longest waiting times. My effort was a rather light-hearted way of underscoring an economics truism: that waiting time may not indicate shortage.

In the same spirit I would like to close this book with another cross-comparison of the fields of restaurants and health care. In this case I take an international perspective. As we have already seen, the WHO ranked the U.S. health care system 37th among 191 nations. Virtually every wealthy nation did better while spending a lower percent of GNP.

As a nation, we do much better with restaurants. To find the world's finest eateries, I consulted the 2007 listing published in *Restaurant* magazine: The S. Pellegrino World's 50 Best Restaurants.[9] As some might expect, France boasts the largest share of the best restaurants, twelve out of fifty. The United States comes in second, with eight top restaurants. The United Kingdom, Spain, and Italy all did well for themselves, with six or seven each. So you could say that the United States had an excellent showing in these rankings. We can surely surmise therefore that Americans in the restaurant field possess talent, attention to detail, business know-how, creativity, and an overarching commitment to excellence. It would be a curious and faulty comparison to suggest that we run our health care system the way we run the restaurant business. The two industries are structured far too differently.

Nevertheless, it can hardly be more obvious that, like the restaurant field, the American health care industry possesses the talent and ingenuity to greatly improve on the cost to outcomes ratio over the next decade. Health systems, medical practices, payers, and purchasers—through the creative application of market incentives—can move steadily toward achieving this goal. There is reason for optimism. Arnie Milstein, for one, envisions a productivity increase that would be the health care equivalent of Moore's Law.[10]

· · ·

I went to the doctor yesterday. He and I have known each other for a long time, and I have great respect for him. We spent most of the visit talking about what he didn't know—the results of my recent diagnostic procedures or even the fact that the procedures had been done. What should have been in the chart was not. So the visit was not an efficient use of time for either of us. As I was about to leave, this dedicated, highly experienced doctor threw his hands in the air in an expression of frustration.

We have to do better. Medicine is too complicated and too important to be this haphazard. It is one thing to pay for efficient medical care, and another to actually receive it. As a patient and as a taxpayer, I pay for medical care to be available—as all Americans do. I want this money to be well spent. I want it to provide the technology and infrastructure that is increasingly necessary. I want it to provide incentives that put quality and efficiency first. I want an integrated workforce that uses teamwork to get the right thing done at the right time. And most of all, I want to know, when the chips are down, that there will be a doctor in the house.

REFERENCE MATTER

APPENDIX A:

THE COST OF TRAINING A DOCTOR

AND THE RETURN ON INVESTMENT

Trained physicians make up the backbone of the health care system. Because of this, the government generally considers it worthwhile to invest in their training. When allocating dollars, policymakers often find it helpful to quantify the specific costs and benefits associated with a particular investment. This appendix provides a structure for thinking about the costs and benefits of training a doctor. It also gives specific estimates, based on a set of assumptions I deemed reasonable.

The analysis indicates that society bears a cost of about $1 million to train a physician. This includes the opportunity cost[1] of forgone wages while the physician spends eight years in training. These costs are spread over an eight-year training period, four years of medical school, and an average of four years of postgraduate training. The rate of return comes from applying these costs to a simple model of return on investment, in which I look at the present value of earnings over a physician's lifetime. Section I provides estimates for the costs of training a physician. It also specifies which stakeholders bear the costs at each stage of the training process. Section II looks at the lifetime rate of return on the investment in a physician's education. All of the estimates have been updated to 2008 dollars.[2]

I. MEDICAL SCHOOL COSTS

The cost of medical school is generally divided into instructional costs and resource costs. Instructional costs are primarily composed of professor salaries and costs that relate directly to the teaching program, whereas total educational resources include all activities of teaching, research, scholarship, patient care, and maintenance of facilities. To obtain an estimate of the cost of medical school, I looked at three sources[3] that estimated the cost of medical school training, and averaged across these sources. To keep the estimate conservative, I used only the instructional costs and excluded the costs of educational resources. Educational resources include other factors, such as the cost of research done by medical students. This gives an estimate of $73,807 for the annual cost of medical school in 2008 dollars.[4]

I estimated the share of medical school costs borne by the government and by medical students, respectively. According to data from the Association of American Medical Colleges, the average medical school charged $28,068 in tuition and fees for the 2006–2007 school year.[5] On the basis of a Florida Board of Governors memo indicating government appropriation per student, I estimated that the government bears 80 percent of the remaining $45,739 after tuition is paid. I believe the rest comes from other sources such as private foundations.

I also took into account the opportunity cost for a medical student to attend school. Specifically, I cared about the foregone wages from spending four years out of the labor force. The 2006 Current Population Survey calculates an average salary of $44,195 dollars for someone with a bachelor's degree between the ages of twenty-five and twenty-nine.[6] The average first-year medical student matriculates at age twenty-four,[7] so I believe this cohort to be representative.

Table A.1 summarizes the annual cost of putting a student through medical school, broken down by stakeholder. The cost to society is simply the sum of

Table A.1. Annual cost of undergraduate medical education in 2008 dollars

	Student	Government	Other	Society (total)
Medical school costs	$28,000	$36,591	$9,148	$73,807
Opportunity cost to student	$44,195	$0	$0	$44,195
Total	$72,263	$36,591	$9,148	$118,002

DATA SOURCES: For inflation adjustment: BLS inflation index CUUR0000SA0. (Please note that all figures have been brought up to 2008 dollars, so they will not be the same as their sources unless the data source reports in 2008 dollars.) For total medical school costs: R. F. Jones and D. Korn, "On the Cost of Educating a Medical Student," Academic Medicine 72, no. 3 (1997): 200–210; American Medical Student Association, www.amsa.org/meded/tuition_FAQ.cfm. For opportunity cost: 2006 Current Population Survey.

the cost to the relevant stakeholders involved. The bottom line is that it costs society about $118,000 dollars a year to train a medical student.

Internship and Residency Costs

As I did with medical school, I estimated the cost of graduate medical education (GME) to different stakeholders: the resident, the hospital, the government, and society.

The cost to the resident (or intern) is the opportunity cost of foregone wages minus the stipend they receive as payment. The Association of American Medical Colleges provides data on the average resident stipend each year past graduation from medical school.[8] My estimates assumed four years of graduate medical education because the modal specialty, internal medicine, requires a one-year internship and three years of residency. Hence, I averaged stipend amounts for the first four years postgraduation to get an average resident stipend of $49,140 in 2008 dollars.

I used two methods to calculate the opportunity cost of graduate training. The methods gave nearly identical results. First, I used the fact that medical school graduates with one year of experience can work in an emergency room. The salary for an emergency room physician with one to four years of experience is $129,626.[9] I therefore assumed an opportunity cost of $44,195 (the same as for medical students) in the first year of GME and then $129,626 thereafter. This gives an average opportunity cost of $114,544. My second method involved using a previously calculated physician wage regression that included "years of experience."[10] This gave me an average opportunity cost of $114,667. For both of these methods, I adjusted for the longer work hours of residents. Residents work 63.6 hours per week, on average, whereas practicing doctors only work 57.8 hours a week. I assumed that the doctor working more hours will make a higher salary at the same hourly rate, and adjusted accordingly. As Table A.2 indicates, the total cost to the resident is equal to $77,032. This reflects the opportunity cost less the resident stipend.

The cost to the government of training a resident depends on Medicare payments. This is complicated by the fact that Medicare's payments for residency can be separated into direct costs and indirect costs, as defined by Medicare. The direct GME payment is based on the number of residents at the hospital, a hospital-specific per-resident amount, and Medicare's share of

Table A.2. Annual cost of graduate medical education in 2008 dollars

	Student	Government	Hospital	Society (total)
Cost				
Opportunity cost for low-experience physician	$126,173			
Medicare payment per resident (paid)		$57,491		
Resident stipend (paid)			$49,140	
Teaching physician slowdown (40% productivity loss * physician salary of $248,912)			$99,565	
Total	$126,173	$57,491	$148,705	$332,369
Value				
Resident stipend (received)	$49,140			
Medicare payment per resident (received)			$57,491	
Nurse practitioner equivalent (69% effective per hour and 1.6 times the weekly hours implies 110% of nurse practitioner salary of $83,190)			$91,214	
Total	$49,140	$0	$148,705	$197,845
Net cost	$77,033	$57,491	$0	$134,524

DATA SOURCES: For inflation adjustment: BLS inflation index CUUR0000SA0. (Please note that all figures have been brought up to 2008 dollars, so they will not be the same as their sources unless the data source reports in 2008 dollars.)

For Medicare payment per resident: MedPAC's "Report to Congress: Rethinking Medicare's Payment Policies for Graduate Medical Education and Teaching Hospitals," August 1999, p. 4; COGME "Fifteenth Report: Financing Graduate Medical Education in a Changing Health Care Environment," December 2000, HRSA; Florida Board of Education, www.flboe.org/BOG.

For nurse practitioner: Salary.com Website http://swz.salary.com/salarywizard/layouthtmls/swzl_compresult_national_HC07000008.html (last accessed Sept. 2007).

For resident stipend: Association of American Medical Colleges Website, www.aamc.org/data/housestaff/hss2006report.pdf (last accessed June 2007).

For physician salary: AMA Socioeconomic Monitoring System data, 1983, 1985, 1987, 1989, 1991, 1993, 1995, 1997, 1999, and 2001.

hospital inpatient days.[11] In addition to this direct payment, Medicare adjusts its standard payment for services depending on how many residents work at a hospital. This is the indirect payment. I obtained estimates of both direct and indirect payments.[12] To keep the estimates conservative, however, I only included the direct cost per resident that Medicare pays to hospitals. Including the indirect cost would have inflated the figure for the cost to the government and deflated the figure for the cost to the hospital. Because I considered all stakeholders with equal weight when calculating the cost to society, my inclusion or exclusion of the indirect Medicare payments would not have an impact on the bottom-line figure of the cost to society of training a doctor. Based on the average of my three sources, the bottom-line estimate of direct Medicare payments per resident physician is $57,491, so that is the GME cost borne by the government.

The hospital's cost of training a doctor may be the most controversial part of this calculation. There are two basic approaches. One school of thought says that the hospital will hire residents up until the point at which the marginal benefit of hiring another resident is equal to the marginal cost of training that doctor. Otherwise, if each new resident brought positive value to the hospital, then the hospital would want to keep hiring more residents. Conversely, if the additional resident costs the hospital, the hospital will not be willing to take on new residents. I will call this the zero-marginal-benefit approach.

The second approach would be to estimate each component of the doctor's value and cost and to add them up. Costs involve paying the resident's stipend, paying doctors to train the resident, and the cost of mistakes the resident makes while learning. The cost to the hospital of doctors to train residents would be the average slowdown of doctors as a result of teaching residents times the doctor's salary. For instance, maybe the doctor experiences a slowdown of 20 percent per resident. If the average doctor salary is $248,912 (from Chapter 3, adjusted into 2008 dollars), then 20% × $248,912 = $99,565.

Benefits to the hospital of having a resident on hand include the Medicare stipend the hospital receives from training the resident and the value of services the resident provides for the hospital. The value of resident services could be estimated using the cost of the closest substitute for a resident. If the hospital didn't have the resident, how would it provide the services that resident normally produces? One way would be to hire a nurse practitioner at $83,190 for a 40-hour work week.[13] The average resident works 63.6 hours a week,[14] or 1.6 times as many hours as an NP. One might assume that residents work more slowly than NPs, because they are learning, in which case, one must guess how productive a resident is per hour compared to an NP. If one believes a resident is 75 percent as productive as an NP, then one would estimate the cost of replacing the resident as 1.6 × 75 percent x $83,190 = $99,204. Residents may be less productive because they take more time to do

Table A.3. Different scenarios of modeling assumptions

	Assumption Methodology (Average Cost)				Zero-Marginal-Benefit Methodology			
	A	B	C	D	E	F	G	H
Cost Assumptions								
Doctor salary	$248,912	$248,912	$248,912	$248,912	$248,912	$248,912	$248,912	$248,912
Teaching slowdown	20%	40%	20%	20%	20%	40%	20%	30%
Teaching cost	$49,782	$99,565	$49,782	$49,782	$49,782	$99,565	$49,782	$74,674
Cost of mistakes	$0	$0	$0	$25,000	$0	$0	$25,000	$25,000
Resident stipend (paid out)	$49,140	$49,140	$49,140	$49,140	$49,140	$49,140	$49,140	$49,140
Value Assumptions								
NP salary	$83,190	$83,190	$83,190	$83,190	$83,190	$83,190	$83,190	$83,190
Ratio of resident hours to NP	1.6	1.6	1.6	1.6	1.6	1.6	1.6	1.6
Productivity per hour (relative to NP)	75%	75%	50%	75%	31%	69%	50%	69%
Implied value of resident's services	$99,204.66	$99,204.66	$66,136.44	$99,204.66	$41,432	$91,214	$66,432	$91,323
Medicare payment per resident (direct)	$57,491	$57,491	$57,491	$57,491	$57,491	$57,491	$57,491	$57,491
Net annual cost to hospital of training resident	–$57,773	–$7,990	–$24,705	–$32,773	$0	$0	$0	$0
Net annual cost to society of training resident	$76,751	$126,533	$109,819	$101,751	$134,523	$134,523	$134,523	$134,523
Total cost of training a doctor	$779,011	$978,141	$911,284	$879,011	$1,010,102	$1,010,102	$1,010,102	$1,010,102

NOTE: Key assumptions highlighted in gray.

DATA SOURCES: For inflation adjustment: BLS inflation index CUUR0000SA0. (Please note that all figures have been brought up to 2006 dollars, so they will not be the same as their sources unless the data source reports in 2006 dollars.)

For government payment: MedPAC's "Report to Congress: Rethinking Medicare's Payment Policies for Graduate Medical Education and Teaching Hospitals," August 1999, p. 4; COGME "Fifteenth Report: Financing Graduate Medical Education in a Changing Health Care Environment," December 2000, HRSA; Florida Board of Education, www.flboe.org/BOG.

For opportunity cost: T. Brown, R. Scheffler, S. Tom, and K. Schulman, "Does the Market Value Racial and Ethnic Concordance in Physician-Patient Relationships?" *Health Services Research* 42, No. 2 (April 2007): 706–726.

For nurse practitioner: Salary.com Website, http://swz.salary.com/salarywizard/layouthtmls/swzl_compresult_national_HC07000008.html (last accessed September 2007).

For resident stipend: Association of American Medical Colleges Website, www.aamc.org/data/housestaff/hss2006report.pdf (last accessed June 2007).

For physician salary: AMA Socioeconomic Monitoring System data, 1983, 1985, 1987, 1989, 1991, 1993, 1995, 1997, 1999, and 2001.

the tasks that they are not familiar with.[15] This would be the value of resident services, given the assumptions imposed in this example. Table A.3 shows how these estimates would vary depending on the assumptions used. The key assumptions are highlighted in the table.

Both approaches to estimating cost to the hospital—the zero-marginal-benefit approach and the assumption approach—have upsides and downsides. On one hand, the assumption approach has too many unknown variables. Assuming my estimates of each component are imperfect, the final estimate could be pretty far off track if I specified incorrectly or left out an important cost.

There is some evidence that the market for residents follows economic incentives, rather than holding strictly to government allocations. Cromwell, Adamache, and Drozd conducted a study of hospitals after the Balanced Budget Act (BBA).[16] The BBA capped the number of residents that the government would support financially. The study found that, four years past the BBA decision, hospitals accepted nearly four thousand residents beyond the allowable payment cap. In addition, the authors calculated a "marginal effective wage" for residents, which is similar to my concept of net cost to the hospital of hiring a resident. The authors report that, "the average marginal effective wage was –$60,000, implying that adding one more resident not only covered all of the resident's fringe loaded stipend but returned over $60,000 in additional revenue as well." These things suggest that the zero-marginal-benefit approach may be a useful tool for estimating, given that economic principles appear to drive the market.

On the other hand, the fact that there is low variance across resident stipends hints that hospitals may not be setting marginal cost exactly equal to marginal benefit when hiring residents. Hospitals pay residents roughly the same amount no matter what specialty they choose, so the variance is low. For a first-year intern or resident, the twenty-fifth percentile of stipends was $41,396 whereas the seventy-fifth percentile was $44,954, and statistics are similar for second-, third-, and fourth-year residents as well.[17] Also, stipends varied by less than 5 percent depending on the type of hospital (state hospitals, nonprofit hospitals, medical schools, and so on), even though these hospitals have different patient mixes and margins of profit. Considering that the variation in physician salaries diverges immediately after residency, the low variance in resident wages indicates that hospitals might not be setting marginal benefit equal to marginal cost when determining the hiring of residents. These indicators suggest that the assumption approach may be more suitable than the zero-marginal-benefit approach.

Ultimately, I chose to use the zero-marginal-benefit approach because of my inability to accurately estimate the many component parameters necessary for the assumption approach. Table A.3 shows some possible ways of breaking down the various components of training a doctor, given the zero-marginal-benefit assumption. Column H, for instance, shows that a 30 percent slowdown in training doctor productivity, a $25,000-per-year cost of resident mistakes, and a 70 percent productivity of residents compared to NPs would yield zero net benefits. Column E shows different assumptions that would also lead to a zero net marginal benefit.

Luckily, the bottom-line figure for the cost of training a doctor does not depend greatly on which approach is used. As Table A.3 shows, the assumption approach implies an $800,000 to $1 million cost of training a doctor. This number would be $1 million under the zero-marginal-benefit approach.

The cost to society of training a resident is equal to the cost of all stakeholders. Table A.2 shows this figure to be $134,523 per year. One oddity of this table is the fact that Medicare payments and resident stipends do not affect the cost to society. This is because Medicare payments are made by the government and received by the hospital. If one weights all stakeholders equally, then this is a wash. The same concept applies to the resident stipend; the hospital pays it and the resident receives it. As a result, the cost to society depends only on the value of the services provided by residents less the teaching slowdown costs and opportunity costs.

Total Cost of Medical Training

Table A.4 summarizes the calculation for the total training costs for each new wave of physicians produced each year in the United States. As discussed in the previous section, I assumed four years of GME for all physicians because that is the number of years required for an internal medicine resident, the modal specialty. General practitioners often take only three years of GME training,[18] but specialist training can range from three to seven years, depending on the specialty.

In 2004–2005, there were a total of 101,291 medical residents.[19] Assuming four years of residency training, on average, there would be 25,323 fully trained physicians entering the workforce each year, costing approximately $13.6 billion in residency training program expenditures. In addition, 15,925 students graduated from medical school in the United States in 2006.[20] This implies a cost of $7.5 billion per year for undergraduate training of a wave of physicians. Not included is the cost of undergraduate training for physicians who did their undergraduate training abroad. About 26.4 percent of U.S. resident physicians come from overseas.[21]

Our figures imply a cost of $1 million for training a physician in the United States. Each new wave of physicians entering the labor force costs society $21.1 billion. Table A.4 depicts the calculations described here. The Veterans Administration trains 1,800 new doctors per year in addition to those who follow the more standard medical education route. Because the training of those doctors follows a different cost structure, they are not included in this cost analysis. However, their presence adds to the costs already included.

The calculation is somewhat sensitive to a few assumptions. For instance, I only included the instructional costs of attending medical school. If the other educational resource costs were added in (about $140,000 extra per year during medical school), this would bring my estimate up to $1.6 million for the total cost of training a doctor. As an economist, I included the opportunity

Table A.4. Costs for training of each new wave of physicians in 2008 dollars

	Cost to Society	Number of Graduates	Total
Four years of medical school	$472,009	15,925	$7.5 billion
Four years of residency	$583,094	25,323	$13.6 billion
Total	$1,010,102	41,248	$21.1 billion

DATA SOURCES: For cost figures: taken from Tables A.1 and A.3 and multiplied by four.

For number of residents: S. E. Brotherton, P. H. Rickey, and S. I. Etzel, "U.S. Graduate Medical Education, 2004–2005: Trends in Primary Care Specialties," *Journal of the American Medical Association* 294, no. 9 (2005): 1075–1082.

For number of medical school graduates: Association of American Medical Colleges Website, http://www.aamc.org/start.htm (last accessed June 2006).

cost. If this were excluded, it would only cost $329,000 in direct costs. My bottom line comes from a set of assumptions and methodologies I believe to be most reasonable.

II. RETURN ON INVESTMENT

I used estimates of the cost of training a doctor to calculate the rate of return to medical education. The methodology follows that of Feldman and Scheffler.[22] Specifically, I calculated the rate of return (ROR) from the following equation,

$$\sum_{t=32}^{65} \frac{B_t - C_t}{(1 + ROR)^{(t-31)}} = 0$$

where B_t is physician earnings once graduating from residency and C_t is the cost of training as calculated earlier. The cost of training does not include the college years, only the medical school years and residency. Assuming an average medical school matriculation age of twenty-four, the resident finishes residency at age thirty-two and practices until the age of sixty-five.

To estimate an earnings profile over the physician's lifetime, I used age coefficients, calculated from American Medical Association data. The distribution of wages across a doctor's lifetime depends on two main factors: the value added from work experience and the depreciation of the doctor's medical education as new techniques replace those he or she learned in medical school. For the first ten years out of residency, the experience factor plays the biggest role. As a result, doctors between the ages of forty-two and fifty-one earn about 16 percent more on average than those below forty-two. However, after the age of fifty-one, the depreciation of the medical education slows down his salary growth. For instance, doctors between fifty-two and sixty-one earn less than one percent more than those in the forty-two to fifty-one age bracket. Older doctors (over sixty-two) actually earn less on average than new doctors out of residency, because their medical education happened so far back in the history of medical advancement.

Using these figures, I calculated that the average return on investment to medical education is about 20 percent. Breaking this figure down into general practitioners and specialists, I found that specialists earn a 22.5 percent return on investment. Assuming only three years of graduate medical education for general practitioners, and accounting for the lower salary, the average GP earns an 18.7 percent rate of return. Interestingly enough, this rate of return is very similar to the rate of return Feldman and Scheffler found thirty years ago.[23] They found a 22 percent rate of return for physicians in 1970.

These figures are quite high compared to the 8.5 percent rate of return on education generally (including high school and college).[24] However, it is reasonable, considering the rate of return for other highly professional degrees. Lawyers earn a 25.4 percent ROR, dentists earn a 20.7 percent ROR, and a graduate business degree will bring about a return of 29 percent.[25]

APPENDIX B:

METHODOLOGY FOR FORECASTING

DOCTOR SHORTAGES[1]

As a baseline for numbers of doctors, we use historical data on physician numbers up to 2001 and projected numbers thereafter assuming that historical trends continue. This gives us a measure of supply. We compare this baseline to two physician-demand forecasts that each employ different methodology. We calculate a needs-based estimate (N) according to the number of doctors that are required to reach the *2006 World Health Report* goal of 80 percent of live births attended by a skilled attendant.[2] The second forecasting approach (D1) reflects the demand for doctors in each country based on projected growth in GNI (gross national income).

The *World Bank Health, Nutrition, and Population Database*[3] gave us a good starting point. This database maintains historical figures on physician numbers and national income (per capita, adjusted for purchasing power parity using the atlas method). I revised these numbers with the most recent figures from WHO for OECD countries.[4] My historical and projected population numbers came from the United Nations Population Division's *2004 Revision Population Database.* Instead of looking at total doctors, I use physician density (per one thousand population). This allows me to account for population growth. My primary indicator for health services provision is the number of live births attended by a skilled health worker.[5] I interpolated data for some countries with missing data. From these data sources, I constructed a panel of 158 countries from 1980 to 2001, grouped according to WHO regional classifications.

For the needs-based approach, I used an arcsine-log model that related physician density with coverage of skilled birth attendants, weighted by population size.[6] This allowed me to identify a level of health worker density below which virtually no country achieved 80 percent coverage. I opted for the arcsine-transformation because it is more consistent with statistical theory. Namely, the transformation of the dependent variable, which is a proportion, results in normally distributed responses (asymptotically).[7] Also, the arcsine-log model showed the highest R^2 and best goodness-of-fit to the data as measured by the deviance. This approach is similar to that followed in the World Health Report.[8]

The economic-based approach utilizes GNI per capita as the predictor of demand for physicians measured per one thousand population with country fixed effects to account for unobservable factors across countries, weighted by population size.[9] Previous research shows that indicators of gross domestic product or national income are the best predictor of health spending.[10] Labor is the principle component of such health care expenditures. I lag GNI per capita by five years. This allowed us to account for the new health care dollars to fully infiltrate the health care system. Because GNI data was only available until 2001, I predicted values of GNI per capita for 2002 to 2010 by assuming past trends would continue forward. My demand equation also included a dummy for the classification of each country by income level (low, medium, and high), based on the World Bank classifications.[11] This allowed me to build into the model the fact that countries with similar levels of development may behave in more similar ways in terms of health care workforce dynamics, and consequently have a different elasticity for physicians.

To compare projections, I classified a country as having a "shortage" if the projected supply meets less than 80 percent of the forecasted demand or need. In addition to the discussion in Chapter 6, Figure B.1 shows graphically how the shortage and surplus distributions play out worldwide. It highlights the problems that Africa faces and the misdistribution across the globe. Table B.1 shows the number of countries in each geographical region with shortages of doctors. Clearly Africa has the largest number of shortages.

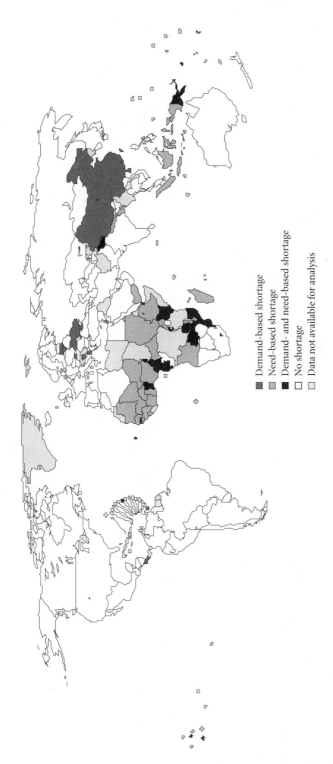

Figure B.1. Global distribution of doctor shortages

NOTE: The boundaries and names shown and the designations used on this map do not imply the expression of any opinion whatsoever on the part of the World Health Organization (WHO) concerning the legal status of any country, territory, city, or area, or of its authorities or concerning the delimitation of its frontiers or boundaries. Dotted lines on maps represent approximate borderlines for which there may not yet be full agreement. (WHO 2007.) All rights reserved.

Legend:
- Demand-based shortage
- Need-based shortage
- Demand- and need-based shortage
- No shortage
- Data not available for analysis

Table B.1. Number of countries with physician shortages in 2015

WHO Region	Needs-Based Model	Economic-Based Model
African	32	15
American	1	3
Eastern Mediterranean	3	2
European	0	10
Southeast Asian	3	0
Western Pacific	6	7
World	45	37

NOTES

CHAPTER 1

1. D. Blumenthal, "New Steam from an Old Cauldron: The Physician-Supply Debate," *New England Journal of Medicine* 350, no. 17 (2004): 1780–1786.

2. In 2001, San Francisco had the largest number of doctors per capita among the fifty largest Metropolitan Statistical Areas in the United States, according to the 2003 Area Resource File, http://sodapop. pop.psu.edu/data-collections/arf/dnd (last accessed April 17, 2008).

3. San Francisco Convention and Visitor's Bureau, "Visitor Facts," www.sfvisitor.org/visitorinfo/html/ VisitorFacts.html (last accessed March 29, 2008).

4. 2004: San Francisco Bay Area Restaurants, Zagat Survey, 2004.

5. "Best Doctors 2005: The Bay Area's 520 Top Docs," *San Francisco Magazine*, January 2005, p. 63.

6. It must be noted that these were not ongoing patient-physician relationships.

7. See note 2.

8. Managed care may also increase the waiting time to see a doctor because enrollees must select from those approved by the managed care firm if they want full coverage.

9. Merritt, Hawkins & Associates, "2004 Survey of Physician Appointment Wait Times," www.merritt-hawkins.com/pdf/mha2004waitsurv.pdf (last accessed March 29, 2008).

10. This estimate includes a conservative estimate of the cost of medical school, an estimate of the net costs of training a resident physician, and the lost wages that the doctor could have made while he or she trains.

11. U. E. Reinhardt, "The Theory of Physician-Induced Demand: Reflections after a Decade," *Journal of Health Economics* 4, no. 2 (1985): 187–193; T. McGuire, "Physician Agency" in *Handbook of Health Economics*, ed. Anthony Culyer and Joseph Newhouse, 461–536 (Amsterdam: North Holland Publishing Company, 2000).

12. A. B. Flood, W. R. Scott, and W. Ewy, "Does Practice Make Perfect? Part II: The Relation Between Volume and Outcomes and Other Hospital Characteristics," *Med Care* 22, no. 2 (1984): 115–125.

13. Definition of *equilibrium:* A market situation that is stable. Nobody wants to adjust their behavior anymore, because they've already adjusted it in response to current market conditions (prices, demand, capacity, and so on).

14. *Washington Sentinel,* "Physician Shortage Points to Healthcare Crisis," American Academy of Emergency Medicine, www.aaem.org/washingtonsentinel/washingtonsentinel_july2006.pdf (last accessed March 29, 2008).

15. Definition of *economic rent:* If you take the lowest amount of money for which someone will provide something and subtract it from what they actually charge, what remains is rent. For example, say doctors are willing to perform a hysterectomy for $400. However, by exercising economic powers, they are able to hike the price up $600. The extra $200 is economic rent.

16. For a more complete history of the supply of physicians, see E. Ginzberg and P. Minogiannis, *U.S. Health Care and the Future Supply of Physicians* (New Brunswick, NJ: Transaction, 2004).

17. A. Flexner, "Medical Education in the United States and Canada," *Bulletin of the World Health Organization* 80, no. 7 (2002): 594–602.

18. R. Fein, *The Doctor Shortage: An Economic Diagnosis* (Washington DC: Brookings Institution, 1967).

19. Ginzberg and Minogiannis, *U.S. Health Care,* 20.

20. Ibid.

21. In 1965 there were approximately eighteen million people in the United States over sixty-five years of age with annual incomes under $1,000 who were unable to afford much medical care before the passage of Medicare and Medicaid. *Source:* Morris Udall, 20th District of Arizona, "Medicare v. Eldercare—A Big Issue Finally Resolved." Congressman's Report, March 31, 1965, Vol. IV, No. 2. Available at www.library.arizona.edu/exhibits/udall/congrept/89th/650331.htm (last accessed March 29, 2008).

22. For an in-depth examination of the political events that led up to and surrounded the Medicare Program, see T. Marmor, *The Politics of Medicare,* 2nd ed. (New York: Aldine Transaction, 2000).

23. Marmor, *The Politics of Medicare.*

24. National Center for Health Statistics, *Health, United States, 2006 with Chartbook on Trends in the Health of Americans,* Hyattsville, Maryland, November 2006, DHHS Publication No. 2006-1232.

25. American Medical Association, *Physician Characteristics and Distribution in the U.S., 2001–2002 Edition* (Chicago: AMA).

26. Graduate Medical Education National Advisory Committee. *Report to the Secretary: Dept. of Health and Human Services. Vol 1, Summary Report.* DHHS Publication No. (HRA) 81-651. Washington, DC: Health Resources Administration, 1986.

27. For example, D. A. Kindig, "Strategic Issues for Managing the Future Physician Workforce," *Baxter Health Policy Review* 2 (1996): 149–182; J. P. Weiner, "Forecasting the Effects of Health Reform on U.S. Physician Workforce Requirement: Evidence from HMO Staffing Patterns," *Journal of the American Medical Association* 272, no. 3 (July 20, 1994): 222–230.

28. For example, S. J. Balla, "Markets, Governments, and HMO Development in the 1990s," *Journal of Health Politics, Policy and Law* 24, no. 2 (1999): 215–238.

29. With the cost of training continuing to increase along with the decline in income, the economic returns to a doctor clearly fell. But it is still a good deal. This is in part because the cost of medical education is highly subsidized by the government.

30. R. M. Scheffler, N. J. Waitzman, and J. M. Hillman, "The Productivity of Physician Assistants and Nurse Practitioners and Health Work Force Policy in the Era of Managed Health Care," *Journal of Allied Health* 25, no. 3 (1996): 207–217.

31. J. P. Weiner, "Prepaid Group Practice Staffing and U.S. Physician Supply: Lessons for Workforce Policy," *Health Affairs Web Exclusive* (2004).

32. Scheffler, Waitzman, and Hillman, "The Productivity of Physician Assistants and Nurse Practitioners."

CHAPTER 2

1. K. J. Arrow, "Uncertainty and the Economics of Medical Care," *American Economic Review* 53 (1963): 941–973; P. Zweifel and W. G. Manning, "Moral Hazard and Consumer Incentives in Health Care," *Handbook of Health Economics* 1B (2000): 409–459.

2. American Medical Association, *Physician Characteristics and Distribution in the U.S.* Department of Data Quality and Measurement, Division of Data and Operations, 2001–2002; and 2005; U.S. Census Bureau. *Statistical Abstract of the United States, 2004–2005.* Available at www.census.gov/prod/www/statistical-abstract-us.html (last accessed March 29, 2008).

3. R. M. Scheffler, "The Potential Impact of Managed Care on the U.S. Health Care Work Force and a New Model for the Delivery of Primary Care," in *Government and Health Systems*, ed. D. Chinitz and J. Cohen (West Sussex, England: John Wiley & Sons, 1998), 350–360; R. M. Scheffler, "Life in the Kaleidoscope: The Impact of Managed Care on the U.S. Health Care Work Force and a New Model for the Delivery of Primary Care," in *Primary Care: America's Health in a New Era*, ed. M. C. Donaldson, K. D. Yordy, K. N. Lohr, and N. A. Vanselow (Washington, DC: National Academy Press, 1996).

4. V. Fuchs, "The Supply of Surgeons and the Demand for Operations," *Journal of Human Resources* 13 (1978): 35–56.

5. See Chapter 1, note 11.

6. R. M. Scheffler, S. D. Sullivan, and T. H. Ko, "The Impact of Blue Cross and Blue Shield Plan Utilization Management Programs, 1980–1988," *Inquiry* 28 (1991): 263–275.

7. Sherry Glied. "Managed Care," in *Handbook of Health Economics*, ed. A. J. Culyer and J. P. Newhouse, vol. 1, 707–753 (Amsterdam: North Holland Publishing Company, 2000).

8. This market is not perfect. Medicare uses the heavy hand of government to set fees for doctors, for example.

9. Hybrid managed care plans such as PPOs and POSs have surpassed HMOs. As of 2001, conventional health plans had 7 percent of the market, HMOs had 23 percent, POSs had 22 percent, and PPOs had 48 percent. *Source:* Jon Gabel, Larry Levitt, Jeremy Pickreign, Heidi Whitmore, Erin Volve, Diane Rowland, Kelly Dhont, and Samantha Hawkins, "Job-Based Health Insurance in 2001: Inflation Hits Double Digits, Managed Care Retreats," *Health Affairs* 20, no. 5 (2001): 180–196.

10. See Chapter 1, note 11; T. McGuire, "Physician Agency," in *Handbook of Health Economics*, vol. 1, ed. Anthony Culyer and Joseph Newhouse, 461–536 (Amsterdam: North Holland Publishing Company, 2000).

11. R. Mayes and R. A. Berenson, Medicare *Prospective Payment and the Shaping of U.S. Health Care* (Baltimore: John's Hopkins University Press, 2006).

12. R. M. Scheffler, "Managed Behavioral Health Care and Supply-Side Economics. 1998 Carl Taube Lecture," *The Journal of Mental Health Policy and Economics* 2, no. 1 (1999): 21–28; M. V. Pauly, "Editorial: A Re-Examination of the Meaning and Importance of Supplier-Induced Demand," *The Journal of Health Economics* 13, no. 3 (1994): 369–372; M. V. Pauly, "The Economics of Moral Hazard: Comment," *American Economic Review* 58 (1968): 531–537.

13. Mayes and Berenson, *Prospective Payment.*

14. One such lawsuit is *Pegram* v. *Herdrich*, 530 U.S. 211 (2000). Cynthia Herdrich, a patient at an HMO, experienced a ruptured appendix after having been told to wait for eight days for an ultrasound after experiencing abdominal pain. She won a malpractice case, but sued her HMO under ERISA, maintaining that the HMO's use of doctors' bonuses was a breach of fiduciary duty. The U.S. Supreme Court denied this, and Justice Souter stated that "No HMO organization could survive without some incentive connecting physician reward with treatment rationing." ("HMOs: Herdrich Survives Charge Against Physician Incentive in High Ct." *Managed Care Week*, June 19, 2000.)

15. D. M. Cutler, M. McClellan, and J. P. Newhouse, "How Does Managed Care Do It?," *The RAND Journal of Economics* 31, no. 3 (2000): 526; R. M. Scheffler, A. B. Garrett, D. A. Zarin, and H. A. Pincus, "Managed Care and Fee Discounts in Psychiatry: New Evidence," *The Journal of Behavioral Sciences and Research* 27, no. 2 (2000): 215–226.

16. D. Emmons and G. Wozniak, "Physicians' Contractual Agreements with Managed Care Organizations," in *Socioeconomics of Medical Practice 1997* (Chicago: American Medical Association, 1997).

17. These changes in hospital admission and length of stay were also the result of the prospective payment system, which was implemented by the Medicare program in 1983.

18. R. M. Scheffler, "United Mine Workers' Health Plan: An Analysis of the Cost-Sharing Program," *Medical Care* 22, no. 3 (1984): 247–254.

19. One caveat: I use HMOs as an example because they are the most consistent measurement of managed care. Unfortunately, although using HMOs as a measure of managed care is quite accurate between 1983 and 1996, after 1996 the number becomes an undercount, because at this time insurance companies began inventing hybrid managed care networks such as PPOs and IPAs—thus between 1996 and 2000 the actual number of managed care organizations was higher than it appears in the chart. So the graph of the percentage of population enrolled in HMOs would actually be steeper than it is in the chart between 1996 and 2000.

20. For example, D. Dranove, C. J. Simon, and W. D. White, "Determinants of Managed Care Penetration," *Journal of Health Economics* 17, no. 6 (December 1998): 729–745. Dranove, Simon, and White examine differences in managed care penetration across geographic areas. They look at the percentage of revenue physicians received from managed care contracts, and rates of enrollment in managed care plans. The authors conclude that demographics, labor market characteristics, and supply-side variables (including the level of concentration in hospital markets, hospital occupancy rates, and the practice organization patterns of physicians) are all important determinants of managed care penetration. On the micro level, a higher per capita concentration of physicians in an area led to greater managed care penetration.

21. J. Gabel, D. Ermann, T. Rice, and G. de Lissovoy, "The Emergence and Future of PPOs," *The Journal of Health Politics, Policy, and Law* 11, no. 2 (1986): 305–322.

22. K. Quinn, *The Sources and Types of Health Insurance* (Boston: Abt Associates, March 1998).

23. Petris Center analysis of the AMA, *Socioeconomic Statistics* (Chicago: American Medical Association, 1983–1995).

24. Petris Center analysis of the American Medical Association *Socioeconomic Statistics* (unpublished private data).

25. S. Glied. "Managed Care," in *Handbook of Health Economics*, vol. 1, ed. A. J. Culyer and J. P. Newhouse, 707–753 (Amsterdam: North Holland Publishing Company, 2000).

26. These figures on HMO penetration at the national level are consistent with the figures in M. S. Marquis, J. A. Rogowski, and J. J. Escarce, "The Managed Care Backlash: Did Consumers Vote with Their Feet?" *Inquiry, the Journal of Health Care Organization, Provision, and Financing* 41, no. 4 (Winter 2004-2005).

27. J. C. Robinson, "Decline in Hospital Utilization and Cost Inflation Under Managed Care in California," *Journal of the American Medical Association* 276, no. 13 (1996): 1060–1064.

28. Data Sources: *National Health Expenditures, 2004* from Centers for Medicare & Medicaid Services, U.S. Department of Health and Human Services; *Health and Aging Chartbook*, Hyattsville, Maryland: National Center for Health Statistics, 1994, 1999, 2003, 2004, and 2005. HMO ($p < 0.00$) and year trend ($p < 0.01$) are both significant predictors of NHE.

29. *The Econ Review*, "President Nixon Imposes Wage and Price Controls," August 15, 1971. www.econreview.com/events/wageprice1971b.htm (last accessed March 29, 2008).

30. Health Care Financing Review, "Hospital Wage and Price Controls: Lessons from the Economic Stabilization Program. (Medicare Payment Systems: Moving Toward the Future)," http://findarticles .com/p/articles/mi_m0795/is_n2_v16/ai_16863001.

31. L. C. Baker and J. C. Cantor, "Physician Satisfaction Under Managed Care," *Health Affairs* 12 Suppl. (1993): 258–270.

32. W. Dow, D. Harris, and Z. Liu, "Differential Effectiveness in Patient Protection Laws: What Are the Causes? An Example from Drive-Through Delivery Laws," *Journal of Health Politics, Policy and Law* 31, no. 6 (2006): 1107–1127.

33. H. S. Luft, *Health Maintenance Organizations: Dimensions of Performance* (New York: John Wiley and Sons, 1981); R. H. Miller and H. S. Luft, "Managed Care Plan Performance Since 1980: A Literature Analysis," *Journal of the American Medical Association* 271, no. 19 (1994): 1512–1519; J. E. Ware, R. H. Brook, W. H. Rogers, E. B. Keeler, A. R. Davies, C. D. Sherbourne, G. A. Goldberg, P. Camp, and J. P. Newhouse, *Health Outcomes for Adults in Prepaid and Fee-for-Service Systems of Care: Results from the Health Insurance Experiment* (Santa Monica, CA: RAND Corporation, 1987).

34. H.R. 1304 was intended "to ensure and foster continued patient safety and quality of care by making the antitrust laws apply to negotiations between groups of health care professionals and health plans and health insurance issuers in the same manner as such laws apply to collective bargaining by labor organizations under the National Labor Relations Act."

35. R. M. Scheffler, "Physician Collective Bargaining in the Era of Managed Care: A Turning Point in U.S. Medicine," *Journal of Health Politics, Policy and Law* 24, no. 5 (1999): 1071–1076.

36. L. P. Casalino, H. Pham, and G. Bazzoli, "Growth of Single-Specialty Medical Groups," *Health Affairs* 23, no.2 (2004): 82–90.

37. Ibid.

38. R. M. Scheffler, "Productivity and Economies of Scale in Medical Practice," in *Health, Manpower, and Productivity*, ed. J. Rafferty (Lexington, MA: Lexington Books, 1974); R. M. Scheffler, "Further Consideration on the Economics of Group Practice: The Management Input," *Journal of Human Resources* 10, no. 2 (1975): 258–263.

CHAPTER 3

1. American Medical Association *Socioeconomic Statistics* (unpublished private data).

2. Board certification is a measure of quality and extra training. A physician who is "board certified" has fulfilled the educational requirements of the field he or she is in and taken a comprehensive written and oral examination given by the certifying board of that specialty.

3. Another way to investigate physician income trends is to differentiate between physicians who work in primary care and those specialists who do not work in primary care. Similarly, we find that both primary care and nonprimary care physicians' incomes increased from 1983 and peaked in 1993. However, incomes for nonprimary care physicians decreased from over $250,000 in 1993 to about $235,000 in 2001, while incomes for primary care physicians remained fairly steady at about $160,000 after 1993. Data source: AMA Socioeconomic Monitoring System data, 1983, 1985, 1987, 1989, 1991, 1993, 1995, 1997, 1999, and 2001.

4. Using standard regression techniques.

5. For details of our analysis, see R. M. Scheffler and J. Liu, "An Analysis of Physician Salaries" (working paper, PETRIS, August 2007).

6. F. A. Sloan and R. Feldman, "Competition Among Physicians," in *Competition in the Health Care Sector: Past, Present, and Future*, ed. W. Greenberg (Washington, DC: Federal Trade Commission, 1978); F. A. Sloan, *Insurance, Regulations, and Hospital Costs* (Lexington, MA: Lexington Books, 1980).

7. J. P. Newhouse, *Pricing the Priceless: A Health Care Conundrum* (Cambridge, MA: MIT Press, 2002).

8. Scheffler and Liu, "An Analysis of Physician Salaries."

9. D. Magrane and P. Jolly, "The Changing Representation of Men and Women in Academic Medicine," *Association of American Medical Colleges: Analysis in Brief* 5, no. 2 (July 2005): 1–2.

10. D. Magrane, J. Lang, and H. Alexander, "Women in U.S. Academic Medicine: Statistics and Medical School Benchmarking 2004–2005" (Washington DC: Association of American Medical Colleges, 2005). Available at www.aamc.org/members/wim/statistics/stats05/wimstats2005.pdf (last accessed March 29, 2008).

11. See note 5.

12. M. B. Rosenthal, B. E. Landon, S. T. Normand, R. G. Frank, and A. M. Epstein, "Pay for Performance in Commercial HMOs," *New England Journal of Medicine* 355, no. 18 (2006): 1895–1902.

13. See page 2 for more discussion.

14. Rosenthal, and others, "Pay for Performance in Commercial HMOs."

15. R. Pear, "Medicare Says It Won't Cover Hospital Errors," *New York Times*, August 19, 2007; J. Rovner, "Medicare to Cut Payments for Avoidable Errors," NPR, August 27, 2007, www.npr.org/templates/story/story.php?storyId=13872687 (last accessed March 29, 2008).

16. M. B. Rosenthal, R. G. Frank, Z. Li, and A. M. Epstein, "Early Experience with Pay for Performance: From Concept to Practice," *Journal of the American Medical Association* 294, no. 14 (October 12, 2005): 1788–1793.

17. M. B. Rosenthal and R. G. Frank, "What Is the Empirical Basis for Paying for Quality in Health Care?" *Medical Care Research and Review* 63, no. 2 (April 2006): 135–157.

18. Rosenthal, and others, "Pay for Performance in Commercial HMOs."

19. Definition of *opportunity cost:* The cost of the next best alternative. When students attend medical school, they are giving up the salaries that they could have made in the workforce. These salaries are their opportunity cost for attending school.

20. I. Walker and Y. Zhu, "The Returns to Education: Evidence from the Labour Force Surveys." Research Report presented to the Department of Education and Skills, no. 313 (University of Warwick, Coventry, West Midlands, United Kingdom, November 2001).

21. R. Feldman and R .M. Scheffler, "The Supply of Medical School Applicants and the Rate of Return to Training," *Quarterly Review of Economics and Business* 18, no. 1 (1978): 91–98.

22. W. B. Weeks, A. E. Wallace, M. M. Wallace, and H. G. Welch, "A Comparison of the Educational Costs and Incomes of Physicians and Other Professionals," *The New England Journal of Medicine* 330, no. 18 (1994): 1280–1286.

23. R. M. Scheffler, R. G. Weisfeld, and E. Estes, "A Manpower Policy for Primary Health Care," *New England Journal of Medicine* 298, no. 19 (1978): 1058–1062.

24. www.medicalhomeinfo.org (last accessed March 29, 2008).

CHAPTER 4

1. R. M. Scheffler, "The Relationship Between Medical Education and the Statewide Per Capita Distribution of Physicians," *Journal of Medical Education* 46 (1971): 995–998.

2. T. Schevitz, "New Med School Part of UC Plan to Boost Health Care Graduates," *San Francisco Chronicle*, November 14, 2006, page B-3.

3. RAND California Community Statistics, "RAND California Population Density in U.S. Counties and Cities," The RAND Corporation, http://ca.rand.org/cgi-bin/homepage.cgi (last accessed March 29, 2008).

4. Area Resource File, 2003, www.arfsys.com (last accessed March 29, 2008).

5. For details, see R. M. Scheffler and J. Liu, "Analysis of Physician Migration Patterns in the U.S. and California" (working paper, PETRIS, 2007).

6. See Chapter 1, note 13.

7. T. T. Brown, J. Coffman, B. Quinn, R. Scheffler, and D. Schwalm, "Do Physicians Always Flee from HMOs? New Results Using Dynamic Panel Estimation Methods," *Health Services Research* 41, no. 2 (2006): 357–373.

8. J. P. Newhouse, "Geographic Access to Physician Services," *Annual Review of Public Health* 11 (1990): 207–230.

9. S. Yeo, "Language Barriers and Access to Care," *Annual Review of Nursing Research* 22 (2004): 59–73; N. Lewin-Epstein, "Determinants of Regular Source of Health Care in Black, Mexican, Puerto Rican, and Non-Hispanic White Populations" *Medical Care* 29 (1991): 543–557; G. X. Ma, "Between Two Worlds: The Use of Traditional and Western Health Services by Chinese Immigrants," *Journal of Community Health* 24 (1999): 421–437; Pew Hispanic Center/Kaiser Family Foundation, *2002 National Survey of Latinos* (Menlo Park, CA). Available at www.kff.org (last accessed April 3, 2005); Morehouse Medical Treatment and Effectiveness Center, "A Synthesis of the Literature: Racial & Ethnic Differences in Access to Medical Care," Kaiser Family Foundation, www.kff.org/minorityhealth/1526–index.cfm (last accessed April 16, 2008).

10. U.S. Census Bureau, "National Population Estimates," *Census 2000 Brief* (March 2001); "*Physician Characteristics and Distribution in the U.S., 2005 Edition*" (Chicago: American Medical Association, 2005). *Note:* Individuals with unknown or missing race or ethnicity information were excluded.

11. T. T. Brown, R. M. Scheffler, S. E. Tom, and K. A. Schulman, "Does the Market Value Racial and Ethnic Concordance in Physician-Patient Relationships?," *Health Services Research* 42, no. 2 (2007): 706–726.

12. Sanofi-Aventis, "2000 eHMO-PPO/Medicare-Medicaid Digest," *Managed Care Digest Series* (2000).

13. J. X. Liu, T. T. Brown, and R. M. Scheffler, "Improving Access to Medical Care for Underserved Minorities: An Analysis of the Supply of Minority Physicians in California," A Study Conducted for the California Program on Access to Care, University of California Office of the President (Petris Working Paper).

14. The numbers may not add up to 100 percent because of rounding and unique racial categorization.

15. Council on Graduate Medical Education, "Tenth Report: Physician Distribution and Health Care Challenges in Rural and Inner-City Areas," U.S. Department of Health and Human Services, February 1998, www.cogme.gov/rpt10.htm (last accessed March 29, 2008).

16. See Chapter 3, note 5.

CHAPTER 5

1. For example, NPs can take patient histories and conduct physicals. R. M. Scheffler, N. J. Waitzman, and J. M. Hillman, "The Productivity of Physician Assistants and Nurse Practitioners and Health Work Force Policy in the Era of Managed Health Care," *Journal of Allied Health* 25, no. 3 (1996): 207–217.

2. R. D. Carter and J. Strand, "Physician Assistants: A Young Profession Celebrates the 35th Anniversary of Its Birth in North Carolina," *North Carolina Medical Journal* 61, no. 5 (2000): 249–256.

3. Ibid.

4. K. L. Grumbach, L. G. Hart, E. Mertz, J. Coffman, and L. Palazzo, "Who Is Caring for the Underserved? A Comparison of Primary Care Physicians and Nonphysician Clinicians in California and Washington." *Annals of Family Medicine* 1, no. 2 (2003): 97–104.

5. Pew Health Professions Commission and the Center for the Health Professions, "Charting a Course for the 21st Century: Physician Assistants and Managed Care." Center for the Health Professions, University of California at San Francisco, http://futurehealth.ucsf.edu/pdf_files/PAexecsum.PDF (last accessed March 29, 2008); E. S. Schneller, recognized for research on the role of physician assistant, received a Robert Wood Johnson Foundation grant in 2004 to track the profession from 1978 to 2000. See some findings at www.rwjf.org/portfolios/resources/grantsreport.jsp?filename=037027.htm&iaid=135 (last accessed March 29, 2008).

6. Career Center: National Student Nurses' Association, "Is Nursing for You?," National Student Nurses' Association, Inc., 2000, www.nsna.org/career/is_nursing_for_you2.pdf (last accessed March 29, 2008).

7. G. D. Sherwood, M. Brown, V. Fay, and D. Wardell, "Defining Nurse Practitioner Scope of Practice: Expanding Primary Care Services," *The Internet Journal of Advanced Nursing Practice* 1, no. 2 (1997), www.ispub.com/ostia/index.php?xmlFilePath=journals/ijanp/vol1n2/scope.xml (last accessed March 29, 2008).

8. M. H. Bowman and K. E. LeRoy, "Physician Supervision in California: Practitioners' Utilization and Perceptions," *Clinical Excellence for Nurse Practitioners* 6, no. 1 (2002).

9. L. E. Berlin and G. D. Bednash, *Enrollment and Graduations in Baccalaureate and Graduate Programs in Nursing* (Washington, DC: American Association of Colleges of Nursing, 2000).

10. A. F. Simon, *Twelfth Annual Report on Physician Assistant Education Programs in the United States, 1995–1996* (Loretto, PA: Physician Assistant Education Association, 1996). For more information, see www.paeaonline.org (last accessed March 29, 2008).

11. R. A. Cooper, "Health Care Workforce for the Twenty-First Century: The Impact of Nonphysician Clinicians." *Annual Review of Medicine* 52 (2001): 51–61.

12. P. D. Jacobson, L. E. Parker, and I. D. Coulter, "Nurse Practitioners and Physician Assistants as Primary Care Providers in Institutional Settings." *Inquiry* 35, no. 4 (1998–1999): 432–446.

13. B. Burkhardt, "You're Sick, We're Quick. An Innovation in Health Care Opens at CVS/Pharmacy Stores in Greater Atlanta—Minute Clinic Provides Quality and Convenience Close to Home and the Workplace," press release, November 7, 2005, www.minuteclinic.com/html/_about/press_room/press_release/CVS_Atlanta_Openings.html (last accessed November 28, 2005).

14. Scheffler, Waitzman, and Hillman, "The Productivity of Physician Assistants and Nurse Practitioners."

15. M. O. Mundinger, R. L. Kane, E. R. Lenz, A. M. Totten, W. Tsai, P. D. Cleary, W. T. Friedewald, A. L. Siu, and M. L. Shelanski, "Primary Care Outcomes in Patients Treated by Nurse Practitioners or Physicians: A Randomized Trial," *Journal of the American Medical Association* 283, no. 1 (2000): 59–68.

16. K. A. Baldwin, R. J. Sisk, P. Watts, J. McCubbin, B. Brockschmidt, and L. N. Marion, "Acceptance of Nurse Practitioners and Physician Assistants in Meeting the Perceived Needs of Rural Communities," *Public Health Nursing* 15, no. 6 (1998): 389–397; W. D. Bottom, "Physician Assistants: Current Status of the Profession," *Journal of Family Practice* 24, no. 6 (1987): 639–644; K. J. Rhee and A. L. Dermyer, "Patient Satisfaction with a Nurse Practitioner in a University Emergency Service," *Annals of Emergency Medicine* 26, no. 2 (1995): 130–132.

17. R. M. Scheffler, "Life in the Kaleidoscope: The Impact of Managed Care on the U.S. Health Care Workforce and a New Model for the Delivery of Primary Care," in *Primary Care: America's Health in a New Era*, ed. M. S. Donaldson, K. D. Yordy, K. N. Lohr, and N. A. Vanselow, 312–340 (Washington, DC: National Academy Press, 1996).

18. Cooper, "Health Care Workforce for the Twenty-First Century."

19. K. E. Martin, "A Rural-Urban Comparison of Patterns of Physician Assistant Practice," *Journal of the American Association of Physician Assistants* 13, no. 7 (2000): 49–50, 56, 59.

20. Cooper, "Health Care Workforce for the Twenty-First Century."

21. Grumbach and others, "Who is Caring for the Underserved?

22. Carle Foundation Hospital, "Carle Telemedicine," www.carle.com/Hospital/centprog/telemedicine.shtml (last accessed March 29, 2008).

23. National Archives and Records Administration, "410.75 Electronic Code of Federal Regulations," http://ecfr.gpoaccess.gov/cgi/t/text/text-idx?c=ecfr;sid=e64d0aa0b745b1d47588482fe66d93a9;rgn=div8;view=text;node=42%3A2.0.1.2.10.2.35.51;idno=42;cc=ecfr (last accessed March 29, 2008).

24. Scheffler, "Life in the Kaleidoscope."

25. J. P. Weiner, "Prepaid Group Practice Staffing and U.S. Physician Supply: Lessons for Workforce Policy," *Health Affairs* Suppl. Web Exclusives (2004): W4–43–59.

26. S. Levine, MD, in discussion with the author, June 13, 2006.

27. Edward O'Neil's essay offers four reasons not to forget this fact. See www.futurehealth.ucsf.edu/from_the_director_0707.html (last accessed March 29, 2008).

28. D. W. Rahn and S. A. Wartman, "For the Health-Care Work Force, A Critical Prognosis," *The Chronicle of Higher Education* 54, no. 10 (November 2, 2007): B14. See also www.bls.gov/oco/cg/cgs035.htm#emply (last accessed March 29, 2008).

29. V. Colliver, "Health Care: It's the Hot Field to Find a Job In," *San Francisco Chronicle*, November 6, 2007, pp. C1, C7. See also www.healthws.com/company/why_workforce.htm (last accessed March 29, 2008).

CHAPTER 6

1. J. P. Weiner, "Prepaid Group Practice Staffing and U.S. Physician Supply: Lessons for Workforce Policy," *Health Affairs* Suppl. Web Exclusives (2004).

2. R. A. Cooper, T. E. Getzen, and P. Laud, "Economic Expansion Is a Major Determinant of Physicians Supply and Utilization," *Health Services Research* 38, no. 2 (2003).

3. See Chapter 1, note 13.

4. Graduate Medical Education National Advisory Committee, Summary Report, DHHS Pub. No. (HRA) 81–651 (Washington, DC: Department of Health and Human Services, 1980).

5. R. M. Scheffler, "Health Expenditure and Economic Growth: An International Perspective," *Occasional Papers on Globalization* 1, no. 10 (University of South Florida Globalization Research Center, November 2004).

6. OECD countries are Australia, Austria, Belgium, Canada, Czech Republic, Denmark, Finland, France, Germany, Greece, Hungary, Iceland, Ireland, Italy, Japan, Korea, Luxembourg, Mexico, Netherlands, New Zealand, Norway, Poland, Portugal, Slovak Republic, Spain, Sweden, Switzerland, Turkey, United Kingdom, and United States.

7. Cooper, Getzen, and Laud, "Economic Expansion Is a Major Determinant."

8. R. E. Hall and C. I. Jones, "The Value of Life and the Rise of Health Spending," *Quarterly Journal of Economics* 122, no. 1 (2007): 39–72.

9. A. Garber, "Editorial: The U.S. Physician Workforce: Serious Questions Raised, Answers Needed," *Annals of Internal Medicine* 141, no. 9 (November 2, 2004): 732–737.

10. Weiner, "Prepaid Group Practice Staffing and U.S. Physician Supply." This paper looks at eight large prepaid group practices—Kaiser Permanente's six regions, Group Health Cooperative of Puget Sound in Seattle, and HealthPartners (HP) in the Twin Cities.

11. R. Scheffler, J. Liu, Y. Kinfu, and M. Dal Poz, "Forecasting the Global Shortages of Physicians: An Economic- and Needs-based Approach" (forthcoming), *Bulletin of the World Health Organization*.

12. Ibid.

13. Directorate for Employment, Labour and Social Affairs Group on Health, "Health Workforce and Migration Study: Preliminary Findings," DELSA/HEA, Dec 21, 2006.

14. B. Guthrie, "P4P: Performing for Pay in UK Primary Care," *Health Affairs*, Aug. 2, 2007, http://healthaffairs.org/blog/2007/08/02/p4p-performing-for-pay-in-uk-primary-care (last accessed March 29, 2008).

15. B. Pond and B. McPake, "The Health Migration Crisis: The Role of Four Organization for Economic Cooperation and Development Countries," *The Lancet* 367, no. 9520 (2006), www.thelancet.com (last accessed March 29, 2008).

16. Ibid.

17. M. B. Forcier, S. Simoens, and A. Giuffrida, "Impact, Regulation and Health Policy Implications of Physician Migration in OECD Countries," *Human Resources for Health* 2, no. 1 (2004): 12.

CHAPTER 7

1. D. Cutler, *Your Money or Your Life: Strong Medicine for America's Health Care System* (New York: Oxford University Press, 2004).

2. See Chapter 1, note 15.

3. J. B. Richmond and R. Fein, *The Health Care Mess: How We Got into It and What It Will Take to Get Out* (Cambridge, MA: Harvard University Press, 2005), 103–104.

4. United States Department of Health, Education, and Welfare, *A Report to the President on Medical Care Prices* (Washington, DC: U.S. Government Printing Office, 1967), in Richmond and Fein, *The Health Care Mess.*

5. Definition of *Zero Sum:* A structure of rewards in which one person's gain is exactly equal to another person's loss.

6. M. E. Porter and E. O. Teisberg, *Redefining Health Care: Creating Value-Based Competition on Results* (Boston: Harvard Business School Press, 2006), 4.

7. R. A. Cooper, "It's Time to Address the Problem of Physician Shortages: Graduate Medical Education Is the Key," *Annals of Surgery* 246, no. 4 (October 2007): 527–533.

8. A. Garber, "Editorial: The U.S. Physician Workforce: Serious Questions Raised, Answers Needed," *Annals of Internal Medicine* 141, no. 9 (November 2, 2004): 732–737.

9. A. M. Rivlin and J. R. Antos, eds., *Restoring Fiscal Sanity 2007: The Health Spending Challenge* (Washington, DC: Brookings Institution Press, 2007), 37.

10. E. Salsberg and A. Grover, "Physician Workforce Shortages: Implications and Issues for Academic Health Centers and Policymakers," *Academic Medicine* 81, no. 9 (September 2006): 782–787.

11. Output is measured in physician salaries.

12. W. B. Weeks, A. E. Wallace, M. M. Wallace, and H. G. Welch, "A Comparison of the Educational Costs and Incomes of Physicians and Other Professionals," *The New England Journal of Medicine* 330, no. 18 (1994): 1280–1286.

13. I. Walker and Y. Zhu, "The Returns to Education: Evidence from the Labour Force Surveys." Research report presented to the Department of Education and Skills, no. 313 (Coventry, West Midlands, United Kingdom: University of Warwick, November 2001).

14. R. Feldman and R. M. Scheffler, "The Supply of Medical School Applicants and the Rate of Return to Training" *Quarterly Review of Economics and Business* 18, no. 1 (1978): 91–98.

15. Porter and Teisberg, *Redefining Health Care: Creating Value-Based Competition on Results,* p. 4.

16. D. Mechanic, *The Truth About Health Care: Why Reform Is Not Working in America* (New Brunswick, NJ: Rutgers University Press, 2006), 17.

17. D. M. Berwick, "My Right Knee," *Annals of Internal Medicine* 142 (2005): 121–125.

18. Rivlin and Antos, *Restoring Fiscal Sanity 2007*, 42–43.

19. Rivlin and Antos, *Restoring Fiscal Sanity 2007*.

20. S. M. Shortell, R. R. Gillies, D. A. Anderson, K. M. Erickson, and J. B. Mitchell, *Remaking Health Care in America: The Evolution of Organized Delivery Systems* (San Francisco: Jossey-Bass, 2000).

21. Institute of Medicine, "Crossing the Quality Chasm: The IOM Health Care Quality Initiative" 2001, www.iom.edu/?id=18795 (last accessed March 29, 2008).

22. E. L. Schneider and J. M. Guralnik, "The Aging of America: Impact on Health Care Costs," *Journal of the American Medical Association* 263, no. 17 (May 2, 1990): 2335–2340.

23. V. Fuchs and E. Emanuel, "Health Care Reform: Why? What? When?" *Health Affairs* 24, no. 6 (November-December 2005): 1399–1414.

24. D. Mechanic, "Physician Discontent: Challenges and Opportunities," *Journal of the American Medical Association* 290, no. 7 (August 20, 2003): 941–945.

25. Cutler, *Your Money or Your Life: Strong Medicine for America's Health Care System*.

26. American Medical Association, *Physician Characteristics and Distribution in the U.S.* (Chicago: American Medical Association, 2006).

27. Educational Commission for Foreign Medical Graduates, ECFMG's 2002 Annual Report, available at www.ecfmg.org/annuals/2002/ (last accessed March 29, 2008).

28. See Chapter 1, note 15.

29. G. D. Sherwood, M. Brown, V. Fay, and D. Wardell, "Defining Nurse Practitioner Scope of Practice: Expanding Primary Care Services." *The Internet Journal of Advanced Nursing Practice* 1, no. 2 (1997), www.ispub.com/ostia/index.php?xmlFilePath=journals/ijanp/vol1n2/scope.xml (last accessed March 29, 2008).

30. V. R. Fuchs, *Who Shall Live? Health, Economics, and Social Choice*, Expanded Edition, vol. 6 (Singapore: World Scientific Publishing Company, 1998).

31. A. Flexner, "Medical Education in the United States and Canada," *Bulletin of the World Health Organization* 80, no. 7 (2002): 594–602.

32. For more information on medical education, see K. M. Ludmerer, *Time to Heal* (New York: Oxford University Press, 1999).

33. BBC News, "Nurses' Role Set To Expand," November 22, 1999, http://news.bbc.co.uk/1/hi/health/527800.stm (last accessed March 29, 2008); L. Barclay, "UK Expands Prescribing Powers for Nurses, Pharmacists," *Medscape Medical News*, November 21, 2005, www.medscape.com/viewarticle/517497 (last accessed April 16, 2008).

34. For more on the use of technology, see A. M. Garber, "To Use Technology Better," *Health Affairs* 25, no. 2 (2006): W51–W53.

35. J. J. Cohen, B. A. Gabriel, and C. Terrell, "The Case for Diversity in the Health Care Workforce," *Health Affairs* 21, no. 5 (September-October 2002): 90–102.

PART II: CONVERSATIONS WITH THE EXPERTS

1. M. E. Porter and E. O. Teisberg, *Redefining Health Care: Creating Value-Based Competition on Results* (Boston: Harvard Business School Press, 2006).

2. A. C. Enthoven and L. A. Tollen, "Competition in Health Care: It Takes Systems to Pursue Quality and Efficiency," *Health Affairs* 24, no. 5 (2005): W5-420–W5-433.

3. K. Davis, et al., "Mirror, Mirror on the Wall: An International Update on the Comparative Performance of American Health Care," The Commonwealth Fund, May 15, 2007, www.commonwealthfund. org/publications/publications_show.htm?doc_id=482678 (last accessed March 29, 2008); The Commonwealth Fund Commission on a High Performance Health System, "Framework for a High Performance Health System for the United States," The Commonwealth Fund, August 2, 2006, www.common wealthfund.org/publications/publications_show.htm?doc_id=387153 (last accessed March 29, 2008).

4. M. Friedman and S. Kuznets, *Income from Independent Professional Practice* (New York: National Bureau of Economic Research, 1945); R. L. Hatzel, "The Contributions of Milton Friedman to Economics," *Economic Quarterly* 93, no. 1 (Winter 2007): 1–30.

5. R. A. Cooper, T. E. Getzen, H. J. McKee, and P. Laud, "Economic and Demographic Trends Signal an Impending Physician Shortage," *Health Affairs* 21, no. 1 (January-February 2002): 140–154.

6. J. P. Newhouse, "Accounting for Teaching Hospitals' Higher Costs and What to Do About Them," *Health Affairs* 22, no. 6 (November-December 2003): 126–129.

7. J. P. Newhouse, "Medicare Spending on Physicians: No Easy Fix in Sight," *The New England Journal of Medicine* 356, no. 18 (May 3, 2007): 1883–1884.

8. J. R. Knickman, M. Lipkin Jr., S. A. Finkler, W. G. Thompson, J. Kiel, "The Potential for Using Non-Physicians to Compensate for the Reduced Availability of Residents" *Academic Medicine* 67, no. 7 (1992): 429– 438.

9. See Chapter 7, note 7.

10. Cooper, Getzen, McKee, and Laud, "Economic and Demographic Trends."

11. David C. Goodman, T. A. Stukel, C. Chang, and J. E. Wennberg, "End-of-Life Care at Academic Medical Centers: Implications for Future Workforce Requirements," *Health Affairs* 25, no. 2 (2006): 521–531; J. E. Wennberg, E. S. Fisher, T. A. Stukel, and S. M. Sharp, "Use of Medicare Claims Data to Monitor Provider-Specific Performance Among Patients with Severe Chronic Illness," October 7, 2004, Web-Exclusive on Health Affairs Website, http://content.healthaffairs.org/cgi/content/full/hlthaff. var.5/DC1 (last accessed March 29, 2008).

12. U. E. Reinhardt, *Physician Productivity and the Demand for Health Manpower: An Economic Analysis* (Cambridge, MA: Ballinger, 1975).

13. Mechanic, *The Truth About Health Care*; J. W. Mold, G. E. Fryer, and A. M. Roberts, "When Do Older Patients Change Primary Care Physicians?," *Journal of the American Board of Family Practice* 17, no. 6 (November-December 2004): 453–460.

14. U. E. Reinhardt, "Planning the Nation's Health Workforce: Let the Market In," *Inquiry* 31, no. 3 (Fall 1994): 250–263.

15. M. B. Rosenthal, R. G. Frank, Z. Li, and A. M. Epstein, "Early Experience with Pay-for-Performance: From Concept to Practice," *Journal of the American Medical Association* 294, no. 14 (2005): 1788–1793.

16. J. Coffman, B. Quinn, T. T. Brown, and R. M. Scheffler, *Is There a Doctor in the House? An Examination of the Physician Workforce in California Over the Past 25 years* (Berkeley, CA: The Nicholas C. Petris Center on Health Care Markets and Consumer Welfare, 2004). Also see http://petris.org/_Archived_ Publications/is_there_a_doctor.htm (last accessed March 29, 2008).

17. http://med.fsu.edu/AboutCOM/default.asp (last accessed March 29, 2008).

18. E. S. Fisher, D. E. Wennberg, T. A. Stukel, D. J. Gottlieb, F. L. Lucas, and E. L. Pinder, "The Implications of Regional Variations in Medicare Spending. Part II: Health Outcomes and Satisfaction with Care," *Annals of Internal Medicine* 138, no. 4 (2003): 288–298.

19. Charles C. Edwards was Assistant Secretary for Health of the U.S. Department of Health, Education and Welfare from 1973 to 1975.

20. J. H. Hibbard, J. Stockard, and M. Tusler, "Hospital Performance Reports: Impact on Quality, Market Share, and Reputation," *Health Affairs* 24, no. 4 (July-August 2005): 1150–1160; A. M. Epstein, "Volume and Outcome: It Is Time to Move Ahead," *New England Journal of Medicine* 346, no. 15 (April 11, 2002): 1161–1164.

21. M. Rosenthal, C. Hsuan, and A. Milstein, "A Report Card on the Freshman Class of Consumer-Directed Health Plans," *Health Affairs* 24, no. 6 (November-December 2005): 1592–1600.

22. E. A. McGlynn, S. M. Asch, J. Adams, J. Keesey, J. Hicks, A. DeCristofaro, and E. A. Kerr, "The Quality of Health Care Delivered to Adults in the United States," *New England Journal of Medicine* 348, no. 26 (June 26, 2003): 2635.

23. E. Litvak, "Managing Unnecessary Variability in Patient Demand to Reduce Nursing Stress and Improve Patient Safety," *Joint Commission Journal on Quality and Patient Safety* 31, no. 6 (June 2005): 330–338.

24. The Research Project Grant (R01) is a grant mechanism used by the National Institutes of Health.

25. J. Zeigler, "Osteopathic Residencies Struggle to Keep Up with the Growing Number of D.O. Grads," *The New Physician*, April 2004, www.amsa.org/tnp/articles/article.cfx?id=103 (last accessed March 29, 2008).

26. T. T. Brown, R. M. Scheffler, S. E. Tom, and K. A. Schulman, "Does the Market Value Racial and Ethnic Concordance in Physician-Patient Relationships?," *Health Services Research* 42, no. 2 (2007): 706–726.

27. For patients over sixty-five across the United States, the average relationship with a primary care physician was about 10.3 years, according to Mold, Fryer, and Roberts, "When Do Older Patients Change Primary Care Physicians?"

28. For a discussion of Medicare subsidies, see J. Cromwell, W. Adamache, and E. Drozd, "BBA Impacts on Hospital Residents, Finances, and Medicare Subsidies," *Health Care Financial Review* 28, no. 1 (Fall 2006): 117–129.

29. R. Feldman and R. M. Scheffler, "The Supply of Medical School Applicants and the Rate of Return to Training," *Quarterly Review of Economics and Business* 18, no. 1 (1978): 91–98.

30. S. A. Schroeder and H. C. Sox, "Internal Medicine Training: Putt or Get Off the Green," *Annals of Internal Medicine* 144, no. 12 (June 20, 2006): 938–939.

31. E. J. Emanuel, "Changing Premed Requirements and the Medical Curriculum," *Journal of the American Medical Association* 296, no. 9 (September 6, 2006): 1128–1131.

32. G. A. Hawker, J. G. Wright, P. C. Coyte, J. I. Williams, B. Harvey, R. Glazier, A. Wilkins, and E. M. Badley, "Determining the Need for Hip and Knee Arthroplasty: The Role of Clinical Severity and Patients' Preferences," *Medical Care* 39, no. 3 (March 2001): 206–216.

33. J. E. Wennberg, E. S. Fisher, J. S. Skinner, and K. K. Bronner, "Extending the P4P Agenda, Part II: How Medicare Can Reduce Waste and Improve the Care of the Chronically Ill," *Health Affairs* 26, no. 6 (2007): 1575–1585, doi: 10.1377/hlthaff.26.6.1575.

34. E. Fisher, D. E. Wennberg, T. A. Stukel, D. J. Gottlieb, F. L. Lucas, and E. L. Pinder, "The Implications of Regional Variations in Medicare Spending. Part I: The Content, Quality, and Accessibility of Care" *Annals of Internal Medicine* 138, no. 4 (2003): 273–287; E. Fisher, D. E. Wennberg, T. A. Stukel, D. J. Gottlieb, F. L. Lucas, and E. L. Pinder, "The Implications of Regional Variations in Medicare Spending. Part II: Health Outcomes and Satisfaction with Care," *Annals of Internal Medicine* 138, no. 4 (2003): 288–298.

35. www.dartmouthatlas.org (last accessed March 29, 2008).

36. I. Morrison and R. Smith, "Hamster Health Care: Time to Stop Running Faster and Redesign Health Care," *British Medical Journal* 321 (2000): 1541–1542.

A FINAL WORD

1. See Part II, note 35.

2. The World Health Report 2000, "The World Health Organization's Ranking of the World's Health Systems," www.photius.com/rankings/healthranks.html (last accessed March 29, 2008).

3. www.cms.hhs.gov/NationalHealthExpendData/downloads/proj2006.pdf (last accessed March 29, 2008).

4. G. C. Halvorson, *Health Care Reform Now!* (San Francisco, Jossey-Bass, 2007).

5. B. Starfield, *Primary Care: Balancing Health Needs, Services, and Technology* (New York: Oxford University Press, 1998).

6. B. Starfield, "The Primary Solution: Put Doctors Where They Count," *Boston Review*, November-December 2005, http://bostonreview.net/BR30.6/starfield.html (last accessed March 29, 2008).

7. Ibid.

8. C. Schoen, R. Osborn, P. T. Huynh, M. Doty, J. Peugh, and K. Zapert, "On the Front Lines of Care: Primary Care Doctors' Office Systems, Experiences, and Views in Seven Countries," *Health Affairs* 25, no. 6 (2006): w555–w571, doi: 10.1377/hlthaff.25.w555. See http://content.healthaffairs.org/cgi/content/full/25/6/w555 (last accessed April 16, 2008).

9. www.theworlds50best.com/ (last accessed March 29, 2008).

10. Moore's Law originated in computer hardware in 1965 when Gordon Moore estimated that the number of transistors that can be inexpensively placed on an integrated circuit would increase exponentially, doubling approximately every two years. The current definition of Moore's Law holds that doubling occurs every eighteen months.

APPENDIX A

1. See Chapter 3, note 19.

2. This adjustment was done using the BLS data series CUUR0000SA0 for CPI inflation adjustment. Because 2007 and 2008 CPI data were not available at the time of this book, we used the June 2007 CPI index as an estimate of the total 2007 CPI, and we estimated the 2008 inflation assuming the same inflation rate as between 2006 and 2007. We used this methodology throughout our calculations.

3. American Medical Student Association Website, www.amsa.org/meded/tuition_FAQ.cfm (last accessed March 29, 2008); R. F. Jones and D. Korn, "On the Cost of Educating a Medical Student," *Academic Medicine* 72, no. 3 (1997): 200–210; L. Franzini, M. D. Low, and M.A. Proll, "Using a Cost-Construction Model to Assess the Cost of Educating Undergraduate Medical Students at the University of Texas, Houston Medical School," *Academic Medicine* 72, no. 3 (March 1997): 228–237.

4. This was estimated using the Higher Education Price Index for inflation. We estimated the 2008 index assuming the same inflation rate as between 2006 and 2007. www.commonfund.org/Templates/Generic/RESOURCE_REQUEST/target.pdf?RES_GUID=EEF9FA9A-85D9–441D-BEC1-E46CAA23E7A7 (last accessed April 16, 2008).

5. Association of American Medical Colleges Website, http://services.aamc.org/tsfreports/select .cfm?year_of_study=2007 (last accessed March 29, 2008).

6. Current Population Survey, Table PINC-04, http://pubdb3.census.gov/macro/032006/perinc/ new04_001.htm (last accessed March 29, 2008).

7. Association of American Medical Colleges Website, www.aamc.org (last accessed March 29, 2008).

8. Association of American Medical Colleges Website, www.aamc.org/data/housestaff/hss2006report .pdf (last accessed March 29, 2008).

9. Payscale.com Website, www.payscale.com/research/US/Job=Physician_%2f_Doctor%2c_

Emergency_Room_(ER)/Salary (last accessed March 29, 2008).

10. T. T. Brown, R. M. Scheffler, S. E. Tom, and K. A. Schulman, "Does the Market Value Racial and Ethnic Concordance in Physician-Patient Relationships?," *Health Services Research* 42, no. 2 (April 2007): 706–726.

11. www.aamc.org/advocacy/library/gme/gme0001.htm (last accessed March 29, 2008).

12. We used an average of three sources. first source: The Florida Board of Education, available at www.flboe.org/BOG (last accessed June 15, 2007); second source: MedPAC's "Report to Congress: Rethinking Medicare's Payment Policies for Graduate Medical Education and Teaching Hospitals" (August 1999, p. 4). We had to use data from Newhouse and Wilensky (2001) to translate these figures into a per-resident direct cost; third source: Council on Graduate Medical Education's "Fifteenth Report: Financing Graduate Medical Education in a Changing Health Care Environment" (December 2000, Health Resources and Services Administration).

13. http://swz.salary.com/salarywizard/layouthtmls/swzl_compresult_national_HC07000008.html (last accessed March 29, 2008).

14. American Medical Association Website, www.ama-assn.org/vapp/freida/spcstsc/0,1238,120,00. html (last accessed March 29, 2008).

15. J. Lave, "The Cost of Graduate Medical Education in Outpatient Settings," in collective volume *Primary Care Physicians: Financing Their Graduate Medical Education in Ambulatory Settings* (Washington, DC: Institute of Medicine, 1989).

16. J. Cromwell, W. Adamache, and E. Drozd, "BBA Impacts on Hospital Residents, Finances, and Medicare Subsidies," *Health Care Financial Review* 28, no. 1 (Fall 2006): 117–129.

17. 2006 *AAMC Survey of Housestaff Stipends, Benefits and Funding*, Autumn 2006 report, updated January 2007, www.aamc.org/data/housestaff/hss2006report.pdf (last accessed March 29, 2008).

18. See note 14.

19. S. E. Brotherton, P. H. Rickey, and S. I. Etzel, "U.S. Graduate Medical Education, 2004–2005: Trends in Primary Care Specialties," *Journal of the American Medical Association* 249, no. 9 (2005): 1075–1082.

20. Association of American Medical Colleges Website, www.aamc.org/start.htm (last accessed March 29, 2008).

21. Brotherton, Rickey, and Etzel, "U.S. Graduate Medical Education, 2004–2005."

22. R. Feldman and R. M. Scheffler, "The Supply of Medical School Applicants and the Rate of Return to Training," *Quarterly Review of Economics and Business* 18, no. 1 (1978): 91–98.

23. Ibid.

24. See Chapter 7, note 13.

25. See Chapter 3, note 22.

APPENDIX B

1. This appendix follows the methodology described in R. Scheffler, J. X. Liu, Y. Kinfu, and M. R. Dal Poz, "Forecasting the Global Shortages of Physicians: An Economic- and Needs-Based Approach," *Bulletin of the World Health Organization* (published online April 3, 2008, at www.who.int/bulletin/volumes/86/07-46474.pdf; paper version).

2. L. Chen, T. Evans, S. Anand, J. I. Boufford, H. Brown, et al., "Human Resources for Health: Overcoming the Crisis," *Lancet*, 364 (2004): 1984–1990.

3. The *World Bank Health, Nutrition, and Population Database* is available to the public at http://devdata.worldbank.org/hnpstats (last accessed March 29, 2008).

4. These OECD physician supply figures reflect only patient care physicians, excluding those individuals who may work in some other capacity, such as administration or research.

5. World Health Organization, *World Health Statistics 2000*.

6. The needs-based model estimates the following equation for all countries i at time t: [arcsine(% coverage$_{i,t}$)] $= \beta_0 + \beta_1{}^*[\ln(\text{Doctors per 1000 population}_{i,t})] + \mu_i + \eta_t + \delta_{it}$. μ and η reflect country and time fixed effects, respectively, and δ is a random error term.

7. J. H. Zar, *Biostatistical Analysis*, 3rd ed. (Upper Saddle River, NJ: Prentice-Hall, 1996).

8. World Health Organization, *World Health Report 2006: Working Together for Health* (Geneva, Switzerland: World Health Organization, 2006), available at www.who.int/whr/2006/whr06_en.pdf (last accessed April 16, 2008).

9. The economics-based model estimates the following relationship: [ln(doctors per 1000 population$_{i,t}$)] $= \gamma_0 + \gamma_1{}^*[\ln(\text{GNI per capita}_{i,t-5})] + \gamma_2{}^*[\text{Income Level}_i] + \mu_i + \zeta_{i,t}$. ζ is the error term. We employ a linear prediction of GNI per capita for each country i at time t for the years 2003 to 2010 for which GNI per capita are not available using the following equation: [ln(GNI per capita$_{i,t}$)] $= \lambda_0 + \lambda_1{}^*[\text{Year}_i] + (\lambda_2{}^*[\text{Year}_i^2]) + \nu_{i,t}$. The quadratic term was only used in prediction if it was significant at a 95 percent confidence level.

10. T. E. Getzen, "Macroeconomic Forecasting of National Health Expenditures," *Advances in Health Economics and Health Services Research* 11 (1990): 27–48.; J. P. Newhouse, "A Model of Physician Pricing," *Southern Journal of Economics* 37, no. 2 (October 1970): 174–183; M. Pfaff, "Differences in Health Care Spending Across Countries: Statistical Evidence," *Journal of Health Politics, Policy and Law* 15, no. 1 (1990): 1–67.

11. The World Bank classifies member economies and all other economies with populations of more than thirty thousand. Economies are divided among income groups according to 2003 gross national income per capita, calculated using the World Bank Atlas method. The groups are as follows: low income, $765 or less; middle income, $766–9,385; and high income, $9,386 or more.

INDEX

AAPA Physician Assistant Census Reports, 57, 58

Adamache, W., 207

Africa: doctor shortages in, 71, 73, 74, 111, 121, 152, 214, 216

African-American doctors, 47, 50, 139, 140–42

age and experience of doctors, 7, 36–37, 183, 210

aging population, 76, 114, 189; chronic disease in, 84, 90, 95, 196; impact on Medicare, 161, 164, 183, 194; and needs-based forecasting of demand for doctors, 65, 66, 67, 74, 84–85; and office visits, 6, 65, 115

American Academy of Pediatrics, 42

American Medical Association (AMA), 188; current recommendation to increase supply of doctors, 158, 162–63, 167; and Physicians For Responsible Negotiation (PRN), 26–27; and retail clinics, 177; supply of doctors restricted by, 107

American Medical Student Association, 202

Americas: doctor shortages in the, 71, 216

Antos, Joseph, 83–84

Arizona: NPs in, 125

As Good As It Gets, 26

Asia: doctors imported from, 73, 111, 121, 152

Asian-American doctors, 48, 50, 51, 139, 141

Association of American Medical Colleges (AAMC), 8, 140, 150, 203, 206

asthma, 193

Atlanta: doctors per capita in, 5; wait times for doctor appointments in, 5

Australia: foreign-trained doctors in, 72; income of doctors in, 73; primary care in, 193; quality of health care system in, 192

Austria: mortality and life-expectancy in, 193; quality of health care system in, 192

autonomy of doctors, 13, 19, 21, 22, 26, 27, 130, 131

baby boomers. *See* aging population

Bakke decision, 140

Balanced Budget Act of 1997, 8, 86, 133, 162, 207

Balla, S. J., 218n28

Barcellona, William J., 184–85

Bazzoli, G., 27

Belgium: mortality and life-expectancy in, 193

Berwick, Don, 186; "My Right Knee," 83

Boston: doctors per capita in, 5, 115; wait times for doctor appointments in, 4, 5

California: anti-affirmative action policies in, 140–41; demand for health workers in, 63; doctors per capita in, 45, 46, 48–49, 217n2; group practice in, 98, 174, 184–85; Hill Physicians in, 185; Hispanics in, 50–51, 139, 141; HMOs in, 48, 60–61; income of doctors in, 48, 49; Integrated Healthcare Association, 105; Medical Board, 127–28; medical schools in, 44; NPs and PAs in, 60–61, 124, 125–26, 127–28, 134; pay for performance in, 105, 173–74, 176, 184; Project Dolce in San Diego County, 127; racial or ethnic distribution of doctors in, 50–51; shortage of doctors in, 185; spatial distribution of doctors in, 45–46; specialty distribution of doctors in, 49–50; supply cycle of doctors in, 16; vs. United States, 45–46, 48–50, 61, 134, 217n2

California Health Care Foundation, 176

Campbell Bill, 26

Canada: foreign-trained doctors in, 72, 152; income of doctors in, 73; mortality and life-expectancy in, 193; primary care in, 193; quality of health care system in, 192

capitation payment, 38, 176; in managed care, 21, 25, 28, 143, 184, 187; in primary care, 96–97; in specialties, 143; in tiered provider networks, 147; virtual capitation, 144

cardiac ablation, 176

Caribbean: doctors exported from the, 72, 152

Carroll, Peter R., 116–19

Casalino, L. P., 27

Caucasian doctors, 48, 50, 51, 76

certified nurse-midwives, 125, 126

chronic care, 59, 78, 105, 179, 183; for aging population, 84, 90, 95, 196; for children, 42; for congestive heart failure, 180, 182, 193; for diabetes, 127, 136, 144, 176, 193; and medical home model, 120, 170, 195; office visits in, 180; relationship to health care expenditures, 193

Civil Right Act of 1964, 140

Clinton health plan, 89

CNAs, 134

Cohen, Jordan J., 120–22, 193

colonoscopies, 175, 177, 178

Commonwealth Fund, 100, 193

community health workers, 155

competition among doctors, 10, 15, 77, 82–83, 97–98, 108, 188; for patients, 7, 13, 19–20, 23, 27, 96, 124

congestive heart failure, 180, 182, 193

Connecticut: doctor-to-population ratio in, 150, 155

Cooper, Richard, 57, 77, 108, 114–15

coronary artery disease: chronic care for, 149, 193; coronary artery bypass surgery, 99, 103, 105, 149

Council on Graduate Medical Education (COGME), 12, 150, 151, 231n12

Cromwell, J., 207

Cuba: doctors exported from, 73

cultural competency/alignment, 151–52, 157

Cutler, David: Your Money or Your Life, 85

CVS pharmacies, 57

Czech Republic: foreign-trained doctors in, 72

Dallas: doctors per capita in, 5; wait times for doctor appointments in, 5

Dal Poz, M. R., 231n1

Dartmouth Atlas, 180, 183, 192

Davis, Karen, 100–103

decision aids for patients, 181–82

Denmark: foreign-trained doctors in, 72; mortality and life-expectancy in, 193; primary care in, 101, 102

Denver: doctors per capita in, 5; wait times for doctor appointments in, 5

depression, 193

Detroit: doctors per capita in, 5; wait times for doctor appointments in, 5

diabetes, 97, 127, 130, 136, 144, 176, 193

disabled children, 42

disease levels, 6, 65, 67

distribution of doctors, racial or ethnic, 45, 47–48, 50–51, 76, 90; ethnic concordance, 50–51, 138–39, 141, 142

distribution of doctors, spatial, 82, 140, 159, 162, 194; California vs. United States regarding, 46, 48–50, 134; differences in doctors per capita, 5, 45, 46, 48–49, 150, 217n2; global distribution, 71–73, 74, 111, 121, 152–53, 213–16, 231n1; impact of doctors' income on, 43–44, 49, 51, 72–73; impact of managed care on, 14, 15, 45–47, 49, 51, 76, 90; as market signal, 9, 191; policies regarding, 43–45; rural areas, 5, 48, 77, 82, 90, 134; suburban areas, 46; vs. supply of doctors, 5; urban areas, 5, 46, 48, 134

distribution of doctors in specialties, 5, 45, 51, 65, 82, 162; in California, 49–50; impact of doctors' income on, 175, 189; impact of managed care on, 47, 49–50, 76; as market signal, 8–9, 34–35, 41, 120, 191; role of government policies in, 86–87, 140

doctors per capita/doctor-to-100,000–population ratio, 5, 11, 19, 65, 115; in California, 45, 46, 48–49, 217n2; vs. demand for services, 78; in Iowa vs. Connecticut, 150; relationship to managed care, 13, 14, 23, 27, 69–70, 220n20

Dranove, D., 220n20

Drozd, E., 207

Eastern Mediterranean: doctor shortages in, 71, 216

economics-based model of demand, 65, 66, 67–69, 70, 71, 74, 213, 214–16, 232n9

Edwards, Charles, 140

Emanuel, Ezekiel, 179

emergency rooms, 203

Enthoven, Alain C., 95–99, 195

Epstein, A. M., 146
equilibrium of supply and demand, 8, 9, 47, 65, 79, 108, 134, 217n13
ERISA, 219n14
Estes, Harvey, 54
Europe: doctor shortages in, 71, 216

faculty members, 56, 63, 141, 157
family practice. *See* general practice / family practice
fee-for-service arrangements, 38, 81–82, 144; vs. managed care, 13, 18–19, 21, 95, 96, 103, 113, 159–60
fees charged by doctors, 6, 7, 9, 38; competition regarding, 10, 13, 77; impact of managed care on, 13, 14, 15, 18–19, 21, 22, 25, 69, 113, 186
Feldman, Roger, 81, 165, 210, 211
Finland: foreign-trained doctors in, 72; income of doctors in, 73; mortality and life-expectancy in, 193
Fisher, Elliott, 131, 182, 186
Flexner Report, 11, 89
Florida: anti-affirmative action policies in, 140–41; Board of Education, 231n12; Board of Governors, 202; medical schools in, 131
forecasts: as aspirational, 188; regarding demand for nonphysician health care workers, 63; with economics-based model of demand, 65, 66, 67–69, 70, 71, 74, 213–16, 232n9; of global demand, 71–73, 74, 213–16; with integrated workforce model of demand, 65, 66, 69–70, 74; with needs-based model of demand, 65, 66, 67, 70, 71, 74, 84–85, 213–16, 232n9; regarding shortage of doctors, 8–9, 68, 71, 74, 78–79, 80, 82, 85–86, 105, 107, 114–15, 165, 166–67, 191–92, 213–16; regarding surplus of doctors, 8–9, 65, 66, 67, 68–69, 70, 74, 78–79, 191–92
France: foreign-trained doctors in, 72, 170; income of doctors in, 73; mortality and life-expectancy in, 193; quality of health care system in, 192
Frank, Richard, 195
Fremd, Tracey O., 123–26
Friedman, M., 107
Fryer, G. E., 229n27
Fuchs, Victor, 19, 89

Geisinger Health System, 102, 103, 187
gender: female vs. male doctors, 29, 33–34, 37–38, 141, 142, 196; relationship to income of

doctors, 33–34, 37–38; relationship to work hours, 29, 37, 196
general practice / family practice, 142, 154–55, 169; board certification of doctors in, 29; cost of training in, 132, 135; GME training for, 208, 210–11; income of doctors in, 30, 31, 32, 33, 34–35, 36, 87, 210–11; return on investment (ROI) for, 41, 80, 210–11
Germany: health care system in, 192, 193; mortality and life-expectancy in, 193; primary care in, 193
Getzen, T. E., 108
Gitnick, Gary, 127–28
global demand for doctors, 16, 71–73, 74, 87, 152–53
GMENAC. *See* Graduate Medical Education National Advisory Committee
Goldmann, Donald, 129–31
Goldsmith, Jeff, 194
government policies: regarding equitable access to health care, 51; financing of doctor training, 6, 8, 11, 86–87, 108, 110, 112, 133, 135, 150, 154, 161–62, 201, 202, 203–5, 206, 208, 218n29, 231n12; financing of PA training, 54–55; regarding health care standards, 87; H.S. 1304, 221n34; impact on supply of doctors, 6, 12, 50, 86–88, 107, 120, 133; managed care regulations, 26; vs. market mechanisms, 6, 83–84; Medicaid payments, 7, 24; Medicare subsidies for residencies, 8, 12, 86–87, 110, 150, 154, 161–62, 203–5, 206, 208, 231n12; regarding NPs, 55, 59, 63, 124, 128; regarding PAs, 54–55, 59, 63
graduate medical education (GME). *See* residents
Graduate Medical Education National Advisory Committee (GMENAC), 11, 12–13, 65, 67
gross national income (GNI), 213, 214, 232n9
Group Health Cooperative of Puget Sound, 225n10
group practice, medical, 97, 117, 167, 221n34; in California, 98, 174, 184–85; and hospitals, 105; and managed care, 27, 96, 98, 184–85, 187, 225n10; NPs and PAs in, 57; and pay for performance, 38, 39–40, 146, 172, 176, 184–85; and primary care, 184; and specialties, 29, 105
Grover, Atul, 132–34
Grumbach, Kevin, 135–36, 193

Halvorson, George: *Health Care Reform Now!*, 193
Harvard University, 140

health care expenditures, 85, 122, 137, 155, 198; for chronic care, 193; impact of managed care on, 14, 22, 23, 24, 25, 27, 168; as percentage of GDP / GNP, 24, 25, 27, 83, 156, 168, 192–93, 197; relationship to growth of economy, 67–69, 74, 114, 168–69, 214; as unsustainable, 104–5, 106

health care system: equitable access to, 51–52, 81–82, 83–84, 138, 189–90, 191–92; industry standards in, 87–89; reform of, 16–17, 82–84, 89–90, 102, 122, 125–26, 163, 189–90, 193, 195; role of trust in, 83, 100, 109, 139, 178. *See also* health care expenditures

Health Care Whack-A-Mole, 177–78, 194

health insurance, 20–21, 90, 96, 97–98, 195; availability of, 16, 67, 83–84, 90, 102, 112, 138; insurance companies, 28, 29; relationship to patient visits, 6; and supplied-induced demand, 19; universal coverage, 83–84, 102, 112, 138. *See also* managed care

health maintenance organizations (HMOs), 96, 114, 167, 184, 187; in California, 48, 60–61; emergence and growth of, 14, 21, 23, 24–25, 219n9, 220n19; PAs and NPs in, 59, 60; pay for performance (P4P) in, 39–40. *See also* Kaiser Permanente; managed care

HealthPartners (HP), 225n10

Health Workforce Solutions, 63

Herdrich, Cynthia, 219n14

Hibbard, J. H., 146

Hillman, J. M., 223n1

Hispanic doctors, 47, 48, 50, 51, 141

hospitalists, 144

hospitals, 38, 146, 148, 167; assumption approach regarding cost of doctor training, 205, 206, 207–8; community hospitals, 160; general hospitals, 177; and GME, 104; and managed care, 20, 21, 22, 26, 30; and medical groups, 105; mortality and frequency of hospitalization, 182–83; NPs and PAs vs. doctors in, 54, 136; and prospective payment, 25, 133, 220n17; and quaternary references, 169–70; specialty hospitals, 177; teaching hospitals, 4, 35, 82, 86, 110, 132, 133, 150, 151, 154, 161, 162, 164, 204, 205, 231n12; zero-marginal-benefit approach regarding cost of doctor training, 205, 206, 207–8

Houston: doctors per capita in, 5; wait times for doctor appointments in, 5

Howard University Medical School, 140

incentives, economic, 51, 84, 197–98; impact on market signals, 13, 18–19, 107–9, 191; and moral hazard, 18–19, 21; related to managed care, 18–19, 21–22, 28, 39–40, 60, 76, 98; related to medical education, 86–87, 107–9, 165, 170, 207; in tiered provider networks, 82, 97, 147–48. *See also* pay for performance (P4P)

income of doctors, 51, 67, 114, 218n29; in California, 48, 49; in hospital-based vs. practice-based specialties, 30, 42, 103; impact of managed care on, 10, 13–14, 15, 19, 21, 22, 25, 29–30, 31, 32, 33–36, 38, 41, 49–50, 59, 76, 89, 108, 113, 186–87; vs. income of all others, 73; as market signal, 9, 13–14, 27, 30, 35, 78–80, 191; for older vs. younger doctors, 210; vs. other professions, 9, 32, 59, 60, 62, 79, 112, 123, 164–65; primary care vs. nonprimary care, 34–35, 41, 79, 101, 103, 111, 130–31, 132, 135–36, 151, 158, 168, 176, 184, 221n3; relationship to age of doctor, 33–34, 36–37; relationship to cost of training, 40–41; relationship to gender, 33–34, 37–38; relationship to industry standards, 87–89; relationship to quality of care, 81–82; relationship to race or ethnicity, 48, 157; relationship to retirement, 166–67; relationship to shortage of doctors, 13–14, 27, 38, 78–79, 88; relationship to spatial distribution of doctors, 43–44, 49, 50, 51, 72–73; relationship to surplus of doctors, 13–14, 27, 38, 78–79, 108, 115, 175; relationship to years in practice, 33–34; in rich countries vs. poor countries, 72–73; role of economic rent in, 9, 76, 87, 88–89, 175, 218n15; specialists' income, 14, 30, 31, 32, 33–35, 41, 79, 101, 103, 111, 123, 130–31, 132, 135–36, 151, 158, 168, 175–76, 189, 210–11, 221n3; top vs. bottom earners, 35–36; trends in, 29–33, 41, 79, 221n3. *See also* pay for performance

independent practice associations (IPAs), 20, 96, 184, 220n19

India: doctors exported from, 73, 111, 121, 152

infant mortality, 193

Institute of Medicine (IOM), 11, 113, 132; Quality Initiative of, 84

integrated care systems, 97–98, 102, 103, 122, 196; defined, 21, 25–26; integrated workforce model of demand, 65, 66, 69–70, 74; NPs and PAs in, 59, 69–70, 74, 95, 158. *See also* health maintenance organizations (HMOs); Kaiser Permanente

international medical graduates (IMGs): in Canada, 72, 152; from Caribbean, 72, 152; from India, 73, 111, 121, 152; in UK, 72–73, 152, 170; in US, 72, 86, 87, 109, 111, 120–21, 150, 151–53, 154, 163, 167, 170–71, 209
internships, 40, 86, 130, 203
Iowa: doctor-to-population ratio in, 155
Italy: quality of health care system in, 192

Japan: income of doctors in, 73; mortality and life-expectancy in, 193; quality of health care system in, 192
joint replacement surgery, 176, 180–81
Jones, R. F., 202

Kaiser Permanente, 188, 225n10; in California, 60–61, 95, 123, 157–60; doctors per capita at, 69–70, 74, 114, 183; hospital costs of, 22; as integrated system, 22, 59, 83, 95, 98, 102, 122, 159–60, 196; language proficiency at, 157; NPs and PAs at, 59, 69–70, 74, 95, 158; preventive care at, 159–60; specialists at, 189
Kindig, D. A., 218n27
Kinfu, Y., 231n1
King, Martin Luther, Jr., 141
Knickman, Jim, 112
Korn, D., 202
Kuznets, S., 107

language proficiency of doctors, 48, 51, 90, 142, 151–52, 155, 157
Latino doctors, 47, 48, 50, 51, 141
Laud, P., 228n5
Lavizzo-Mourey, Risa, 137–39
lay health coaches, 144
leaders / managers: doctors as, 188–89
Lee, Philip R., 140–42
life-expectancy: in United States vs. other countries, 193
Litvak, Eugene, 148
Liu, J. X., 231n1
Los Angeles: doctors per capita in, 5; hospitals in, 182; mortality rate in, 182; vs. Sacramento, 182; supply of doctors in, 134, 182; wait times for doctor appointments in, 5
loss-and-replacement scenario, 67

malpractice liability insurance, 4, 166
managed care: admissions review in, 20; backlash against, 15, 22, 26–27, 113, 168, 187, 191, 219n14; bonuses for doctors in, 22; capitation payment in, 21, 25, 28, 143, 184, 187; decline of, 15, 25, 49–50, 113, 191; defined, 20–21; doctor-managed care organization contracts in, 20, 21, 24, 27, 28; emergence and growth of, 9, 10, 13–15, 18–20, 23, 24–25, 29, 41, 47, 53, 76, 77, 114, 168–69, 186–87, 220n20; vs. fee-for-service, 13, 18–19, 21, 95, 96, 103, 113, 159–60; and group practice, 27, 96, 98, 184–85, 187, 225n10; impact on autonomy of doctors, 13, 19, 21, 22, 27, 130; impact on doctor-patient relationship, 100–101; impact on fees charged by doctors, 13, 14, 15, 18–19, 21, 22, 25, 27, 28, 69, 113, 154, 168, 186–87; impact on health care expenditures, 14, 22, 23, 24, 25, 27, 168; impact on hospitals, 20, 21, 22, 26, 30; impact on income of doctors, 9, 10, 13–14, 15, 19, 21, 22, 25, 29–30, 31, 32, 33–36, 38, 41, 49–50, 59, 76, 89, 108, 113, 186–87; impact on nurse practitioners, 9, 10, 14–15, 53, 59, 60–61, 76; impact on out-patient vs. inpatient care, 21, 22, 133; impact on physician assistants, 9, 10, 14–15, 53, 59, 60–61, 76; impact on quality of care, 14, 22, 26, 143; impact on racial and ethnic distribution of doctors, 76; impact on spatial distribution of doctors, 14, 15, 45–47, 49, 51, 76, 90; impact on specialties, 22, 23, 29–30, 31, 32, 33–36, 41, 47, 49–50, 76; impact on specialty distribution of doctors, 47, 49–50, 76; impact on wait times, 4, 217n8; market signals under, 9, 13–14, 19–20, 51, 53, 69, 115, 191; relationship to surplus of doctors, 8–9, 13, 23, 27, 67, 76, 108, 154, 220n20; second opinions in, 20, 22, 23. See also health maintenance organizations (HMOs); independent practice associations (IPAs); point-of-service organizations (POSs); preferred provider organizations (PPOs)
marketplace: cartel-inspired contrived scarcity, 107, 108, 109; and equitable access to health care, 51–52, 83–84; global demand for doctors, 16, 71–73, 74, 87, 152–53; vs. government, 6, 83–84; and industry standards, 87–89; market-clearing situations, 6; market pressure, 9, 76; and physician supply cycle, 10–16; and social goals, 51–52; supplier-induced demand, 19, 21, 108, 113, 115
market signals: impact of economic incentives on, 13, 18–19, 107–9, 191; income of doctors, 9, 13–14, 27, 30, 35, 78–80, 191; under managed care, 9, 13–14, 19–20, 51, 53, 69, 115, 191; rate of return on training, 9,

40–41, 80–81; of right number of doctors,
8–10; of shortage, 13–14; students' specialty
preferences, 9, 34–35, 41, 120, 191; of surplus, 13–14; and turning points, 8–9
Mayo Clinic, 95, 105, 183, 187, 188
MCAT scores, 165
McGlynn, Beth, 147
McKee, H. J., 108
measurement of performance, 144, 174, 176,
188, 190; Medicare's policy on avoidable
errors, 137–38; and patient decision aids,
181–82; public disclosure, 98–99, 116, 173,
195; and tiered provider networks, 82–83,
146–48. *See also* pay for performance
Mechanic, David, 83, 115
Medicaid, 36, 59, 218n21; Centers for Medicare &
Medicaid Services (CMS), 110, 130, 137–38,
181, 182, 192–93; and chronic care, 127; fee
schedule, 7, 24; impact on supply of doctors,
11, 107; pay for performance in, 173–74
medical assistants, 134, 136
medical errors, 183
medical home model, 42, 100, 102, 103, 113, 129;
and chronic care, 120, 170, 195
medical schools: AAMC, 8, 140, 150, 203, 206; African Americans in, 140–42; AIDS programs
in, 142; allopathic vs. osteopathic, 121–22,
156, 163, 170; Asians in, 51, 141; available
slots in, 10, 11, 64, 77, 87, 88, 109, 133, 142,
150, 151, 154–55, 158–59, 165, 166, 195; in
California, 44; cost of training in, 130–31,
140, 201–3, 208–9, 217n10; instructional
costs for, 201–2; policies regarding affirmative action in, 140–41; pool of applicants,
154–55, 165; relationship to distribution of
doctors, 43–44; resource costs for, 201–2;
student preferences regarding specialties,
9, 34–35, 41, 120, 169–70, 191; teaching of
research skills in, 88; tuition in, 202; women
in, 141. *See also* training of doctors
Medicare, 36, 138, 218n21; Advantage plans,
103; aging population's impact on, 161, 164,
183, 194; Centers for Medicare & Medicaid
Services (CMS), 110, 130, 137–38, 181, 182,
192–93; fee schedule / relative value scale, 7,
25, 111, 118, 162, 169, 173, 219n8; financing
of residents / GME by, 8, 11–12, 86, 110–11,
118, 135, 150, 161, 164, 203–5, 208, 231n12;
impact on supply of doctors, 11–12, 90, 107,
120; MedPac (Medicare Payment Advisory
Commission), 104, 110, 164, 204, 206,
231n12; pay for performance under, 173,

180, 182; payment of NPs under, 59; policy
regarding avoidable errors, 137–38; prospective payment under, 25, 133, 220n17
Meharry Medical College, 140
Merritt, Hawkins & Associates, 4, 79
Miami: doctors per capita in, 5; supply of doctors in, 183; wait times for doctor appointments in, 4, 5
military health care, 54, 89, 176–77
Milstein, Arnold, 143–48, 194, 197
Minneapolis: doctors per capita in, 5; wait times
for doctor appointments in, 5
Mold, J. W., 229n27
Moore's Law, 145, 197, 230n10
moral hazard, 22; managed care vs. fee-for-
service regarding, 18–19, 21
Morrison, Ian, 186–90, 194; on "Hamster Health
Care," 186
mortality: avoidable deaths, 156; in cardiac
cases, 159–60; relationship to frequent use
of supply-sensitive care, 182–83; in United
States vs. other countries, 193
Mullan, Fitzhugh, 149–53

National Institutes of Health, 229n24
need estimates, 19, 183; needs-based model of
demand, 65, 66, 67, 69, 71, 74, 84, 108, 213,
214–16, 232n6
neonatal mortality, 193
Netherlands, the: mortality and life-expectancy
in, 193; primary care in, 193
Newhouse, Joseph P., 110–11, 231n12
New York City: supply of doctors in, 5, 134, 183;
wait times for doctor appointments in, 4, 5
New York State: bypass graft surgery in, 99;
medical education in, 162, 164
New Zealand: foreign-trained doctors in, 72;
primary care in, 193
Nixon, Richard, 25
nonphysician health care workers, 85, 86, 144,
191, 194, 196; growth in number of, 56, 57,
60–63, 78; service overlap with doctors, 15,
17, 53–54, 56–57, 60–61, 123–24, 128; substitution for doctors by, 9, 54, 60–63, 69–70,
79, 112, 118, 133–34, 165, 175, 178–79. *See
also* certified nurse-midwives; medical assistants; nurse practitioners (NPs); physician
assistants (PAs)
North Dakota, 102, 103
number of doctors: benchmark for "right"
number, 8, 10, 14, 17, 33, 76–78, 78–80,
108, 191, 192; vs. nonphysician health care

workers, 56, 61–63, 69; in primary care, 101, 120, 131, 151, 159, 162, 163, 169, 189, 193, 195; relationship to quality of care, 76–77, 131, 155–56, 192; in specialties, 9, 17, 163, 169, 189, 193; in U.S., 3, 10, 64–65. *See also* distribution of doctors, spatial; distribution of doctors in specialties; doctors per capita / doctor-to-100,000–population ratio

nurse practitioners (NPs): emergence of, 10, 53, 58; in group practice, 57; impact of managed care on, 9, 10, 14–15, 59, 60–61, 76; impact on demand for doctors, 9, 10, 15, 17, 56–57, 60–61, 63, 65, 69–70, 74, 78, 125–26, 133–34, 165; income of, 55–56, 58, 59, 60, 112, 118, 123, 136, 158, 204, 205, 206; and integrated workforce model of demand, 65, 69–70, 74; at Mayo Clinic, 95; and Medical Practice Act, 124, 128; number of, 56, 57, 60–61, 78; and prescription writing, 54, 55, 125, 128, 134; in primary care, 85, 102, 123, 136; productivity of, 7, 57, 59, 61, 69–70, 78, 112, 165, 204, 205, 206, 208; quality of care provided by, 59, 124–25, 127–28; relations with doctors, 55, 57, 124, 125, 128; safety issue regarding, 124–25, 127–28; services performed by, 15, 17, 53–54, 56–57, 60–61, 63, 79–80, 85, 88, 102, 112, 118, 123–26, 127–28, 133–34, 136, 149, 165, 185, 223n1; in specialty care, 53–54, 56, 85, 123–24, 149; training of, 55, 56, 134, 165; in underserved areas, 59

nurses: demand for, 63, 108; income of, 55–56; number of, 55, 56; in primary care, 136; services performed by, 55–56, 85, 134, 136, 144, 175, 177; staffing ratios, 155–56; training of, 55, 56, 103, 109, 113; Transforming Care at the Bedside Project, 129; in UK, 90

office visits: in chronic care, 180; doctors vs. NPs and PAs regarding, 57, 59, 123–24; of elderly patients, 6, 65, 115; and electronic schedule templates, 123–24; length of, 28–29, 115, 185; number of, 6, 67, 114–15, 129–30, 185

O'Neil, Edward, 63, 154–56

Oregon: Greenfield Clinic in, 134

Organization for Economic Cooperation and Development (OECD), 67, 170, 213, 232n4; member countries, 225n6

osteopathy, 121–22, 154, 156, 163, 170

outpatient care, 21, 22, 133

oversupply of doctors. *See* surplus of doctors

Pacific Business Group on Health, 146

Palo Alto Medical Clinic, 189

patient education, 181–82, 195, 196

Pauly, Mark V., 107–9, 191

pay for performance (P4P), 98–99, 144–46, 190; in California, 105, 173–74, 176, 184; in chronic care, 182; and group practice, 38, 39–40, 146, 172, 176, 184–85; impact on specialties, 116–17, 184–85; incentive size, 113–14, 172, 173; level of reward, 172, 176; in Medicare, 173, 180, 182; and preference-sensitive care, 180–82; in primary care, 39–40, 42, 72–73, 103, 184–85; relationship to quality of care, 38–40, 137–38, 144–45, 172, 195; in specialty care, 116–17, 184–85; thresholds of quality vs. improvement over time, 172; types of incentives, 173; in United Kingdom, 38, 72–73, 111

Pearl, Robert, 157–60, 196

Pegram v. Herdrich, 219n14

Pennsylvania: Geisinger Health System, 102, 103, 187

Petris Center, 126

Pham, H., 27

Philadelphia: doctors per capita in, 5; wait times for doctor appointments in, 5

Philippines: doctors exported from, 73

physician assistants (PAs): emergence of, 10, 53, 54, 58, 89, 177; in group practice, 57; impact of managed care on, 9, 10, 14–15, 59, 60–61, 76; impact on demand for doctors, 9, 10, 15, 17, 56–57, 60–61, 63, 65, 69–70, 74, 78, 125–26, 133–34; income of, 55–56, 58, 59, 60, 112, 136, 158; and integrated workforce model of demand, 65, 69–70, 74; number of, 56, 57, 60–61, 78; and prescription writing, 54, 55, 125, 128, 134; in primary care, 54, 55, 85, 136, 149; productivity of, 7, 57, 59, 61, 69–70, 78, 112, 165; quality of care provided by, 59, 124–25, 127; relations with doctors, 54, 55, 57, 59, 124, 125, 128; safety issue regarding, 124–25, 127; services performed by, 15, 17, 53–54, 55, 56–57, 59, 60–61, 63, 79–80, 85, 88, 89, 112, 124–26, 127–28, 133–34, 136, 149, 165, 224n5; in specialty care, 56, 85, 149, 158; training of, 54–55, 56, 134, 165; in underserved areas, 54–55, 59

Physicians For Responsible Negotiation (PRN), 26–27

Pizzo, Philip A., 161–63

point-of-service organizations (POSs), 20, 219n9

Porter, Michael, 82–83, 97–98

Portland, Or.: doctors per capita in, 5; wait times for doctor appointments in, 5

preference-sensitive care, 180–82, 192

preferred provider organizations (PPOs), 20, 24, 25, 96, 187, 219n9, 220n19

prescription writing, 54, 55, 56, 88, 101, 102, 125, 128, 134

preventive care, 97, 118, 136, 159–60, 195, 196

primary care, 11, 179, 229n27; capitation payment in, 96–97; centrality of, 42; and chronic care, 42; defined, 34; in Denmark, 101, 102; gatekeeper model, 189; GME training for, 208; and group practice, 184; income of doctors in, 34–35, 41, 79, 101, 103, 111, 130–31, 132, 135–36, 151, 158, 168, 176, 184, 221n3; internal medicine, 29, 30, 31, 32, 33, 34, 132, 142, 169, 170, 203, 208; and language proficiency of doctors, 48, 157, 158; medical assistants in, 136; medical home model in, 42, 100, 102, 103; vs. non-primary care, 34–35, 41–42, 44, 47, 48, 79, 80, 85, 87, 115, 120, 132, 135–36, 149, 151, 154–55, 158, 163, 168, 169–70, 184–85, 189, 193, 194, 208, 211–12, 221n3; NPs in, 85, 123, 136, 156; number of doctors in, 101, 120, 131, 151, 159, 162, 163, 169, 189, 193, 195; osteopaths in, 156; PAs in, 54, 55, 85, 136; patient-doctor relations, 44, 48, 157, 158, 229n27; pay for performance (P4P) in, 39–40, 42, 72–73, 103, 184–85; pediatrics, 29, 30, 31, 32, 33, 34, 178; racial or ethnic distribution of physicians in, 47–48, 141, 142, 157; in United States vs. other countries, 193. *See also* general practice / family practice; specialties

productivity: of doctors, 7, 57, 59, 61, 62–63, 65, 77–78, 84–85, 112, 130, 143, 148, 159, 165, 178, 185, 189, 195, 204, 205, 207, 208; of nurse practitioners, 7, 57, 59, 61, 69–70, 78, 112, 165, 204, 205, 206, 208; of physician assistants, 7, 57, 59, 61, 69–70, 78, 112, 165; and technology, 7, 85, 86, 90, 178, 194, 195

profiling of providers, 144–45, 146

prospective payment, 25, 133, 145, 220n17

quality of care, 6, 67, 106, 197–98; in chronic care, 137; competition regarding, 77, 82–83; with fee-for-service, 18; with managed care, 14, 22, 26, 143; and pay for performance, 38–40, 137–38, 144–45, 172, 195; provided by NPs and PAs, 59, 124–25, 127–28; relationship to income of doctors, 81–82;

relationship to language proficiency, 48, 51, 90, 157; relationship to measurement of performance, 82–83, 113–14, 145, 146–47; relationship to number of doctors, 76–77, 131, 155, 192; in tiered provider networks, 82–83, 96–97, 146–48

quality of doctors: quality distribution, 81–82; vs. quality of restaurants, 3–4, 35, 82, 197; relationship to doctors' experience, 7; relationship to wait times for appointments, 3–4

Reinhardt, Uwe E., 112–15, 173, 195

rent, economic, 9, 76, 87, 88–89, 175, 218n15

Research Project Grant, 229n24

residents, 44, 121–22, 162; available slots for, 64, 133, 150, 154, 158–59, 170–71, 188, 195; cost of residency programs, 40, 77, 104–5, 110–11, 112, 118, 133, 135, 150, 161–62, 164, 201, 203–10, 217n10, 231n12; in foreign countries, 142; income of, 112, 164–65, 205, 207–8; medical students' choice of specialties, 34–35, 41; Medicare subsidies for residency positions, 8, 11–12, 86–87, 110, 150, 154, 161–62, 203–5, 206, 208, 231n12; work hours of, 112, 136, 203, 205

restaurants: bills evenly shared at, 18, 19; high income doctors vs., 36; quality in United States vs. other countries, 197; quality of doctors vs. quality of, 3–4, 35, 82, 197; supply of doctors vs. supply of, 3–4, 6, 35, 197

retirement of doctors, 165–67, 196

return on investment (ROI): for dental graduates, 41, 80, 107, 211; for doctors, 9, 40–41, 80–81, 107–8, 164–65, 201, 210–11, 218n20; for education in general, 41, 81, 211; for graduate business degrees, 41, 80, 81, 211; for law graduates, 41, 80, 81, 164–65, 211; as market signal, 9, 40–41, 80–81; for training of doctors, 9, 40–41, 80–81

rheumatoid arthritis, 127

Rivlin, Alice, 83–84

Roberts, A. M., 229n27

Robert Wood Johnson Foundation, 129, 224n5

Rosenthal, Meredith, 146–47

rural areas: doctors in, 5, 48, 77, 82, 90, 134; NPs in, 95; PAs in, 59

Sacramento, 182

safety: and Health-Care-Whack-A-Mole, 177–78; and substitution for doctors, 178–79

salary payment, 38

Salsberg, Edward S., 164–67, 196

San Diego: doctors per capita in, 5; wait times for doctor appointments in, 5
San Francisco: Health Workforce Solutions in, 63; supply of doctors in, 4, 134, 197, 217n2; supply of restaurants in, 3–4, 82, 197; wait times for doctor appointments in, 4
Schneller, E. S., 224n5
Schroeder, Steven, 168–71
Seattle: doctors per capita in, 5; wait times for doctor appointments in, 4, 5
SF-36 health survey, 145
shortage of doctors, 65, 189; in Africa, 71, 73, 74; defined, 6, 107; Flexner Report on, 10; forecasts of shortage, 8, 68, 71, 74, 78–79, 80, 82, 85–86, 105, 107, 114–15, 165, 166–67, 191–92, 213–16; market signals for, 13–14, 27, 41, 78–89; in 1960s, 11, 15; and PA movement, 54–55; relationship to income of doctors, 13–14, 27, 38, 78–79, 88; surplus as preferable to, 85–86, 194–95
Shortell, Stephen M., 84, 172–74, 195
Simon, C. J., 220n20
Smith, Mark D., 175–79, 194
Smith, Richard: on "Hamster Health Care," 186
social goods: doctors as, 6, 14; vs. economic units, 14, 31
Souter, David, 219n14
Southeast Asia: doctor shortages in, 71, 216
Sox, Harold, 170
Spain: mortality and life-expectancy in, 193; quality of health care system in, 192
specialties: anesthesiology, 29, 30, 32, 33, 79, 175; board certification, 29, 34, 221n2; capitation payment in, 143; cardiology, 4, 5, 123, 132, 149, 159–60, 180; dermatology, 4, 5; differences in board certification, 29; differences in cost of training, 132; differences in doctors per capita, 5; differences in income, 14, 30, 31, 32, 33–35, 41, 79, 123; differences in wait times for appointments, 4, 5; distribution of doctors in, 9–10, 45, 47, 49–50, 51, 65, 76, 82, 86–87, 140, 162, 175, 189; gastroenterology, 175, 177, 178; and group practice, 29, 105; hospital-based vs. practice-based, 30; impact of managed care on, 22, 23, 29–30, 31, 32, 33–36, 41, 47, 49–50, 76; income of doctors in, 14, 30, 31, 32, 33–35, 41, 79, 101, 103, 111, 123, 130–31, 132, 135–36, 151, 158, 168, 175–76, 189, 210–11, 221n3; internal medicine, 29, 30, 31, 32, 33, 34, 132, 142, 169, 170, 203, 208; lack of ethnic and racial diversity in, 139; medical students' choice of,

34–35, 41; and Medicare, 12; NPs and PAs in, 53–54, 56, 60, 85, 123–24, 149, 158; number of doctors in, 17, 189, 193; ob/gyn, 4, 5, 30, 31, 32, 33, 79, 123, 155; orthopedic surgery, 4, 5, 149, 176, 181–82; pathology, 30, 31, 32; pay for performance in, 116–17, 184–85; pediatrics, 29, 30, 31, 32, 33, 34, 178; psychiatry, 29, 30, 31, 32, 33, 79, 151–52, 169, 178; radiology, 29, 30, 31, 32, 33, 79, 169, 175; radiotherapy, 169; return on investment (ROI) for, 41, 210–11; surgery, 4, 5, 22, 23, 30, 31, 32, 33, 36, 44, 47, 48, 79, 81–82, 116–17, 149, 150, 155, 158, 160, 176, 180–81, 183. *See also* distribution of doctors in specialties; general practice/family practice; primary care
spinal devices, 176
Stanford University: affirmative action policies at, 140, 142; School of Medicine, 142, 163
Starfield, Barbara, 193
substitution for doctors, 79, 175, 178–79; by NPs and PAs, 9, 60–61, 69–70, 112, 118, 133–34, 165
supply cycle of doctors, 10–16; in California, 16; forecasts regarding, 15, 17, 75–76; impact of technology on, 75
supply-sensitive care, 180, 182–83
Supreme Court: *Pegram v. Herdrich*, 219n14
surplus of doctors, 3, 64–65; defined, 6; forecasts of surplus, 8, 65, 66, 67, 68–69, 70, 74, 78–79, 191–92; impact of surpluses, 6–7, 85–86, 154, 194–95; market signals for, 13–14, 27, 41, 78–79; in 1980s, 11, 12–13; as preferable than shortage, 85–86, 194–95; relationship to income of doctors, 13–14, 27, 38, 78–79, 108, 115, 175; relationship to managed care, 9, 13, 23, 27, 67, 76, 108, 154, 220n20; relationship to Medicare, 12–13
Sweden: foreign-trained doctors in, 72, 170; mortality and life-expectancy in, 193
Switzerland: foreign-trained doctors in, 170

team-based care, 7, 78, 85, 89, 90, 95, 129, 184–85, 189, 195
technology, 16, 152; electronic medical records, 101–2, 113, 136, 159, 185, 196; email use, 127, 185; impact on supply cycle of doctors, 17, 75, 90; information technology (IT), 78, 86, 95, 96, 97, 101–2, 117, 129, 159, 160, 165, 195; and productivity, 7, 85, 86, 90, 178, 194, 195; specialists' control of, 175; in *Star Trek* vs. *Star Trek: Voyager*, 75; telemedicine, 90, 127, 177, 185

Teisberg, Elizabeth Olmsted, 82–83
Texas: anti-affirmative action policies in, 140–41
tiered provider networks, 82–83, 96–97, 146–48
Tollen, Laura, 97–98
training of doctors: cost of training, 6, 40–41, 69, 77, 87–88, 109, 130–31, 132, 140, 156, 164, 165, 191–92, 201–11, 217n10, 218n29; course of study, 179, 187; depreciation of medical education, 210; educational debt, 118–19, 130, 135, 169, 170; foundation financing, 11, 202; government financing, 6, 8, 11, 86–87, 108, 110–11, 112, 118, 133, 135, 150, 154, 161–62, 164, 201, 202, 203–5, 206, 207, 208, 231n12; industry standards in, 87–89; length of time for, 120; opportunity cost, 40, 201, 202, 203, 206, 209, 217n10, 222n19; rate of return on, 9, 40–41, 80–81, 107–8, 164–65, 201, 210–11. *See also* medical schools; residents
Transforming Care at the Bedside Project, 129
treatments and cures: coronary artery bypass surgery, 99, 103, 105, 149; innovation in, 67, 120–21; joint replacement surgery, 176, 180–81
trends: in board certification, 29; in gender of doctors, 37; in health care expenditure, 27; in income of doctors, 29–33, 41, 79, 221n3; in income of NPs and PAs, 58, 59; in number of nonphysician health care workers, 56, 57, 60–63, 78; relationship to market signals, 9; in retirement of doctors, 166–67; vs. turning points, 8
trust, 83, 100, 109, 139, 178
turning points: decline of managed care, 15, 25, 49–50, 113, 191; emergence of managed care, 9, 10, 13–14, 18–20, 23, 29, 41, 47, 76, 77, 114, 168–69, 186–87, 220n20; and market signals, 9; vs. trends, 8

underserved areas, 51, 127, 151; NPs and PAs in, 59; and poverty, 85–86, 188; rural areas, 5, 48, 59, 77, 82, 90, 95, 134
unions, physician, 26–27
United Kingdom: distribution of doctors in, 45; foreign-trained doctors in, 72–73, 152, 170; medical schools in, 130; mortality and life-expectancy in, 193; nurses in, 90; pay for performance in, 38, 72–73, 111; primary care in, 72–73, 130–31, 193; quality of health care system in, 192
United Nations Population Division: *2004 Revision Population Database*, 213

United States: vs. California, 45–46, 48–50, 61, 134, 217n2; foreign-trained doctors in, 72, 86, 87, 109, 111, 120–21, 150, 151–52, 154, 163, 167, 170–71, 209; mortality and life-expectancy in, 193; vs. other countries, 16, 45, 73, 101–2, 104, 130–31, 137, 192–93, 197
University of California, Berkeley: Goldman School of Public Policy, 88
University of California, San Francisco, 117, 118, 140–41, 142
University of North Carolina in Chapel Hill, 43–44, 109
University of Washington, 142

Veterans Administration, 122, 209
Virginia Mason, 188

wait times for doctor appointments: and managed care, 4, 217n8; relationship to supply of doctors, 3–4, 82, 197; vs. waiting times for restaurant reservations, 3–4, 197
Waitzman, N. J., 223n1
Washington, D.C.: number of doctors in, 115; wait times for doctor appointments in, 5
Washington State: anti-affirmative action policies in, 140–41; NPs in, 125
Weiner, Jonathan P., 12, 14, 114, 218n27, 225n10
Wennberg, John E., 115, 180–83, 186, 192
Western Pacific: doctor shortages in, 71, 216
White, W. D., 220n20
Wilensky, Gail, 104–6, 195, 231n12
Wisconsin: Healthy Wisconsin, 96; Marshfield Clinic, 95, 98; pay for performance in, 173
work hours of doctors: gender differences, 29, 37, 196; number of hours devoted to nonpatient care, 28, 29; number of hours per week, 6, 7, 29, 35, 36, 37, 112, 126, 136, 166, 167, 203, 205; number of patients seen, 28, 123; in residencies, 112, 136, 203, 205; shift work, 29, 135, 169; weeks worked per year, 28, 29, 35
work hours of NPs and PAs, 112, 136, 204, 205
World Bank classifications of countries by income level, 214, 232n11
World Bank Health, Nutrition, and Population Database, 213, 231n3
World Health Organization (WHO), 71, 192, 213, 215
World Health Report of 2006, 213, 214

Yale University, 140

zero-sum game, 77, 226n5